GUT HEALTH SIMPLIFIED!

7 PROVEN HACKS TO MAKE PEACE WITH FOOD, ACHIEVE MENTAL CLARITY, AND IMPROVE YOUR OVERALL HEALTH FROM THE INSIDE OUT!

LIAM D. CONNAUGHT

Copyright © 2024 - Liam D. Connaught - All rights reserved.

The content within this book may not be reproduced, duplicated, or transmitted without direct written permission from the author or the publisher.

Under no circumstances will any blame or legal responsibility be held against the publisher, or author, for any damages, reparation, or monetary loss due to the information contained within this book, either directly or indirectly.

Legal Notice:

This book is copyright protected. It is only for personal use. You cannot amend, distribute, sell, use, quote, or paraphrase any part of the content within this book, without the consent of the author or publisher.

Disclaimer Notice:

Please note the information contained within this document is for educational and entertainment purposes only. All effort has been expended to present accurate, up-to-date, reliable, and complete information. No warranties of any kind are declared or implied. Readers acknowledge that the author is not engaged in the rendering of legal, financial, medical, or professional advice. The content within this book has been derived from various sources. Please consult a licensed professional before attempting any techniques outlined in this book.

By reading this document, the reader agrees that under no circumstances is the author responsible for any losses, direct or indirect, that are incurred as a result of the use of the information contained within this document, including, but not limited to, errors, omissions, or inaccuracies.

TABLE OF CONTENTS

About the Author   5
Introduction   7

1. GUT HEALTH 101   11
   Gut Health: The Foundation of Your Well-Being   11
   Understanding the Digestive System   12
   The Gut–Brain Connection Demystified   14
   Your Gut Health   18
   The Fantastic World of Your Gut Microbiota   20
   Common Gut Issues Unraveled   25

2. HACK #1: BOTTOMS UP   31
   Hydrate Your Way to a Happy Gut   31
   Hydration and Gut Health   32
   How Much Water Should You Be Drinking?   37
   Water-Rich Foods for Hydration   40
   Are All Beverages Created Equal?   42

3. HACK #2: BOOST YOUR GUT HEALTH WITH FIBER   45
   The Importance of Fiber   45
   Fiber and Gut Health   46
   How Much Fiber Should You Be Eating?   48
   Types of Fiber: Soluble vs. Insoluble   49
   The Risks and Signs of Too Much Fiber   51
   My Tips for Incorporating More Fiber Into Your Diet   51
   Increase Your Fiber Intake—But Gradually   55
   Dos and Don'ts for Increasing Your Fiber Intake   57

4. HACK #3: NOURISH YOUR GUT   61
   A Balanced Diet for Optimal Digestion   61
   Check Your Diet   62
   Choose Whole Foods   67
   Mindful Eating   75

5. HACK #4: CHILL OUT — 81
   Reduce Stress and Improve Sleep for a Happier Gut — 81
   How Stress Affects Gut Health — 83
   Benefits of Stress Management Techniques for Gut Health — 87
   Tips for Managing Stress — 89

6. HACK #5: MOVE IT — 107
   How Exercise Can Improve Your Gut Health — 107
   How Movement Affects Gut Health — 108
   Exercises to Support Your Gut Health — 110
   Tips for Making Your Exercise Routine More Gut-Friendly — 112
   Overcoming Barriers to Exercise — 113

7. HACK #6: GIVE IT A BREAK — 117
   Intermittent Fasting for a Happy Gut — 117
   The Problem With Snacking and Late-Night Eating — 118
   Understanding Intermittent Fasting — 119
   Benefits of Intermittent Fasting for Gut Health — 121
   Getting Started With Intermittent Fasting — 122
   Setting Yourself Up for Intermittent Fasting Success — 127

8. HACK #7: FUEL UP — 131
   Supplementing Your Gut — 131
   Overview of Dietary Supplements — 132
   Choosing a Supplement to Support Your Gut Health — 134
   Tips for Incorporating Supplements in Your Daily Life — 136

   Conclusion — 141
   References — 145

ABOUT THE AUTHOR

The complexity of gut health, frequently overlooked by people and their healthcare providers, has driven me to write with a passion as vibrant as the bustling community of microorganisms in a well-cared-for gut.

The inspiration behind this book stems from my own experiences and a strong desire to help others avoid the health challenges that have affected my dear family and friends. My family's medical history is like a gripping medical drama, filled with conditions like depression, irritable bowel syndrome, thyroid issues, multiple sclerosis, Alzheimer's disease, and cancer. These battles have fueled my curiosity, pushing me to explore the connections between our food choices, gut health, chronic disease, and longevity. I have spent a lot of time unraveling these connections. With this book, I aim to demystify them for you and showcase the transformative power of nurturing our bodies from the inside out.

I want to help you overcome digestive problems, prevent the onset of chronic illnesses, stay out of the doctor's office, and live a long and healthy life. I strongly advocate for evidence-based holistic approaches that harmonize diet and lifestyle changes, guiding us toward a more natural path to healing.

I envision a future where the guidance of nutritional knowledge replaces the clinical approach to medical procedures. In this future, individuals are empowered to actively manage their gut health and create a more fulfilling and healthier life. With this book, I aim to guide you toward this brighter future. This is a story of hope, resilience, and the gut health revolution.

If you consider yourself "well read" on all matters of gut health, then this book might not be for you. However, if this is your first stop with the subject, or if you have attempted to understand what gut health is about but have found it to be a somewhat complex and difficult-to-grasp topic, then you are in the right place! My goal is to spare you from wading through numerous medical journals or endless testimonials that may only cover one aspect of gut health. While this field may be new to many, much has already been written recently on the topic, often targeted toward specific demographics or types of readers. I aim to make this information accessible, relevant, and easy to understand for everyone while providing seven straightforward yet effective hacks to follow.

Although I will include important references to the scientific and academic literature for further reading on all of the topics covered, my primary objective is simplicity—explaining the medical facts and outlining the steps that you can take to improve your gut health or assist a friend or family member in doing so.

As you embark on this journey that will forever change how you understand and care for your gut, get ready to uncover the secrets that will empower you to take charge of your overall well-being. Together, we will explore the fundamental principles and practical strategies that simplify the complex world of gut health.

INTRODUCTION

Uncomfortable digestive symptoms interfere with the daily lives of nearly 40% of the American population (Reed, 2022). If this sounds familiar, you will understand the constant struggle of bloating, constipation, diarrhea, indigestion, reflux, and pain. You will also know that for many people, everyday activities we often take for granted, such as exercising, running errands, and spending time with loved ones, become difficult because of these symptoms. Even more concerning is that many of those who suffer from gut health issues are too embarrassed to seek help.

Our gut health plays a central role in our overall well-being. Have you ever known someone whose health problems felt like a perplexing mystery? Perhaps a family member, a friend, or even yourself? They may have struggled with repeated episodes of bloating, abdominal cramping, and unpredictable bowel movements that had effects far beyond their gut, leaving them feeling fatigued and frustrated.

Like countless others in similar situations, they may have sought answers from various doctors and alternative practitioners, only to find themselves trapped in a confusing maze of tests and consultations.

Days may have turned into weeks, weeks into months, and months into years, yet the elusive root cause of their health issues remained out of reach. With each passing day, their resilience may have been tested while their hope for a resolution began to fade.

But just when they were on the verge of giving up, a glimmer of hope might have emerged. Through careful observation and experimentation, they may have discovered a connection between specific dietary choices and their health, eventually resulting in a diagnosis of irritable bowel syndrome or another gut issue (and IBS is just one of many). For many people, this breakthrough moment marks the beginning of a transformative journey.

By making deliberate adjustments to their eating habits and lifestyle, identifying and avoiding trigger foods, incorporating more soluble fiber in their diet, staying well hydrated, and managing their stress levels, many individuals in this situation gradually begin to feel positive effects throughout their body. Their symptoms of constipation, bloating, and abdominal pain begin to subside and be replaced by renewed energy and improved well-being.

Aspects of this story may resonate with someone close to you, or perhaps they reflect your own experiences. As you seek answers, understanding the challenges faced by individuals dealing with gut issues and the profound impact that gut health can have on one's life may offer the insight and inspiration you are looking for.

So, if you are like me and searching for ways to improve your gut health while reducing your risk of heart disease, dementia, thyroid disease, and cancer, know that you are in the right place. All too often, people wait until their symptoms worsen and they reach a point of desperation before seeking help. Let this book be your guide to achieving a healthier body and a well-balanced gut.

I understand your confusion and curiosity about gut health, as well as your yearning for relief if you are among the large number of people suffering from bothersome symptoms. You may have been down this road before, seeking help from doctors only to face the same dismissal repeatedly. It is frustrating and disheartening. I am honored to share with you seven proven gut health hacks that will transform your relationship with food, provide you with a balanced and nutritious diet, stabilize your gut microbiota, and ultimately unlock the door to the healthiest version of yourself.

Now, picture yourself saying goodbye to the days of feeling exhausted, anxious, and stressed because of digestive problems, allowing you to no longer be at the mercy of your unpredictable gut. Instead, imagine a vibrant life where you regain control, savor each bite of food with confidence, and radiate with vitality. At first, breaking free from daily stomach discomfort may seem like a daunting task, but get ready for a revolution in gut health. This book presents a comprehensive and holistic approach to enhancing the health of your gut and overall body. You will develop tools to get to the root of your gut-related issues, leading to a happier and healthier gut that supports your overall well-being. From reading this book, you can expect a range of incredible benefits that will leave you feeling optimistic about your journey with gut health:

- Improved digestion: Bid farewell to digestive troubles.
- Increased energy: Say goodbye to chronic fatigue and sluggishness.
- Mental clarity: Unlock your mind's potential with enhanced focus and sharper thinking.

- Reduced stress and anxiety: Experience a sense of calm as your gut health improves.
- Better sleep: Prepare for nights of restorative sleep.
- Enhanced immune system: Strengthen your body's defenses and stay healthy.
- Better quality of life: Embrace each moment fully and live life joyfully.

So, let us embark on this transformative journey. Together, we will unravel the mysteries of the gut, discover the secrets and practical steps that will lead you to a healthier body, and rewrite your story. Your gut health transformation begins now!

NOTE: The sources cited in the body of this book and listed in the References section at the end are intended as further reading if you wish to examine in more detail some of the key points made in that part of the text, as researched and discussed in the medical and scientific arena.

1

GUT HEALTH 101

GUT HEALTH: THE FOUNDATION OF YOUR WELL-BEING

 "All disease begins in the gut."

— HIPPOCRATES

Although he said this over 2000 years ago, it turns out that Hippocrates may have been onto something (Harkins et al., 2021). Your gastrointestinal system, including your stomach, small intestine, and colon, is much more than a long tube for the digestion of food. It is critical to your overall health and well-being (Shurney, 2019).

Your gastrointestinal system obviously plays an essential role in digestion and nutrient absorption, but did you know it also affects your immune system, metabolism, and mental health? In other words, gut health is the captain that steers your health ship.

This chapter will lay the foundations for understanding gut health and its impact on your overall health. We will explore the anatomy and functions of the digestive system, dive into the incredible world of the gut microbiota, and uncover how gut health influences your entire body. We will also discuss common gut-related issues that affect millions of people worldwide.

UNDERSTANDING THE DIGESTIVE SYSTEM

To demystify gut health, we first need to understand the anatomy and functions of the digestive system. It is a complex network of organs and processes that break down food, absorb nutrients, and manage waste.

Your food begins its journey in the mouth, from which it enters the digestive system by passing down the esophagus to the stomach, where it is churned up into a puree. From there, it goes into the small intestine, where most of the digestion and absorption of nutrients happens, and finally to the large intestine or colon, which is responsible for water absorption and waste management (Ogobuiro, n.d.).

Let us now take a closer look at each pit stop along the digestive journey:

Mouth: Chewing your food breaks it into smaller pieces and mixes it with enzyme-containing saliva, allowing it to be swallowed.

Esophagus: The esophagus is the muscular tube that moves food from your mouth to your stomach after swallowing.

Stomach: When the food enters your stomach, it is churned into a paste and mixed with stomach acid and enzymes, breaking it down into smaller particles and simpler molecules.

Small intestine: The small intestine is where most of the magic happens. The pureed food from the stomach encounters an array of digestive enzymes that further break down the ingested food to release nutrients, which are absorbed into the bloodstream.

Colon (large intestine): The colon is responsible for the absorption of water and some remaining nutrients. The leftover indigestible parts of food are then prepared for elimination.

Rectum and anus: Finally, the food waste passes out of your body through the rectum and anus.

Several other organs also play important roles in the digestion of food and absorption of nutrients. They include the following:

Liver: Bile is a water-based fluid produced in the liver that is essential for breaking down fats.

Gallbladder: The bile made by the liver is stored in the gallbladder before being released into the small intestine to help digest fats.

Pancreas: The pancreas lies behind the stomach and produces enzymes vital for the digestion of proteins, fats, sugars, and starches in the small intestine. This elongated organ also releases hormones that regulate your appetite, stimulate stomach acid production, and control the emptying of your stomach into the small intestine. It is also responsible for neutralizing the highly acidic stomach contents as they pass into the small intestine, which is essential for protecting the intestinal lining and allowing digestive enzymes to function optimally.

All of the organs in the digestive tract work together in a carefully choreographed series of muscle contractions and biological and chemical reactions. They could not perform their functions without the secretion of numerous crucial enzymes and hormones, as outlined below.

Digestive enzymes: Many enzymes are involved in the digestion of your food. Each plays a unique role in breaking down specific molecules that make up the food you eat. They work behind the scenes, gradually disassembling your food into manageable parts. For instance, lipases are responsible for breaking down fats, amylases digest starches, and proteases dissect proteins and peptides. Without these enzymes, the sugars, amino acids, fatty acids, vitamins, and minerals in your food would not be released for absorption into your blood to support cellular processes throughout your body.

Digestive hormones: Hormones are chemical messengers that work throughout your body and tell your organs what they must do. Gastrin, for example, instructs your stomach to prepare for food breakdown by releasing gastric juices. Cholecystokinin is like a conductor, ensuring your gallbladder releases bile for fat digestion and prompting the pancreas to send in more enzymes. These hormones, along with many others, work hand-in-hand with digestive enzymes to make sure everything runs smoothly.

THE GUT–BRAIN CONNECTION DEMYSTIFIED

Your gut and brain are like friends who have not seen each other for a while but have never lost touch. It may sound strange, but there is a strong link between the two, and it all began when you were a tiny embryo. They developed from the same place, forming a connection that shapes your body's functions. The gut–brain connection is a complex network of nerves, hormones, and other messengers that ensures constant communication between them (Rutsch et al., 2020).

The Enteric Nervous System (ENS)

Imagine the enteric nervous system (ENS) as a tiny "mini-brain" in your gut. This remarkable system controls gut functions independently without involving your brain. It comprises a network of cells called neurons spanning your throat to your bottom. It oversees crucial gut processes like digestion and moving food along the gastrointestinal tract by stimulating the muscle contractions known as peristalsis.

The ENS plays several vital roles in the digestion of food. First, it controls the contractions of the muscles that move food through the gut. Second, it regulates the release of stomach acid. Its third function is stimulating the secretion of digestive hormones, and finally, the ENS influences the immune system in the gut.

If there is a problem in your digestive tract, this efficient web of nerves will sense it and communicate the issue to your brain through a specialized nerve called the vagus nerve. In this way, the ENS keeps your brain updated on what is happening in your gastrointestinal system.

But here is the exciting part: the ENS and the brain are engaged in an ongoing two-way conversation. Your brain sends signals to the ENS to control gut functions, and the ENS sends feedback about the current situation in the gut to the brain.

The Link Between Gut Health and Mental Health

If the gut talks to the brain and the brain talks to the gut, you may wonder whether there is a link between gut health and mental health. While this remains a rapidly evolving topic of scientific research, there is indeed a connection between the two (Xiong et al., 2023).

You already know that the vagus nerve acts as the superhighway connecting the gut and the brain and that the ENS is a critical part of the digestive system. However, they have other functions too. One of them is to make and release essential neurotransmitters such as serotonin and dopamine, which are well known for their roles in regulating your mood.

In addition, the friendly bacteria living in your gut are also involved in synthesizing these important chemicals, giving us an intriguing clue as to why gut disorders can cause mood disorders and vice versa. We will talk more about these microbes later in this chapter.

As such, your gut, intestinal microorganisms, and nervous system work together as a team to keep your body and mind in tip-top shape. When your gut is in harmony, your brain follows suit, and you experience good health and well-being.

The gut–brain connection is a captivating world where your gut and brain are best friends, constantly communicating and influencing each other. Your ENS and gut microorganisms are the unsung heroes in ensuring that everything runs smoothly. As you will discover, this connection plays a crucial role in not only your digestive health but also your mental well-being. Some of the mental health conditions where it is believed to have an impact are presented below.

Anxiety

The neurotransmitters produced in your gut are mood regulators, influencing your emotions and how you feel. Serotonin, for example, is often referred to as a "feel-good" chemical. It may surprise you that 95% of the serotonin in your body is made in your gut (Banskota et al., 2019). Accordingly, when your gut is in good shape, it keeps serotonin production running smoothly and contributes to your overall well-being.

However, serotonin production may be interrupted when things are out of equilibrium due to poor gut health, an imbalance in intestinal bacteria, or inflammation. The resulting drop in serotonin levels may lead to symptoms of anxiety.

Other essential characters in this story include gamma-aminobutyric acid and dopamine, which are also neurotransmitters that affect how you feel.

Depression

Imagine your gut as a bustling city, with tiny microbial citizens managing your mood. These citizens, collectively referred to as the gut microbiota, are key players in producing and releasing special chemicals that are closely tied to your emotions, such as serotonin and dopamine. However, when the balance of the gut microbiota gets disrupted (a state we call "dysbiosis"), it can throw off the levels of these brain chemicals. This can lead to inflammation and disrupt communication between your gut and brain, potentially making you feel depressed.

Brain Fog

Have you ever experienced brain fog? It feels like a cloud settling over your mind, making it hard to concentrate, remember, and think clearly. One of the likely culprits behind brain fog is chronic inflammation in the gut, which can trigger an immune response. This immune response releases inflammatory molecules called cytokines that can sneak into your bloodstream and cross the blood–brain barrier. Once in your brain, they can interfere with brain function and contribute to brain fog (Fernández-Castañeda et al., 2022).

An imbalance in the gut microbiota can result in the production of toxic chemicals such as lipopolysaccharides, which can impair cognitive function and memory. In other words, when your gut is not happy, it can make your brain feel a bit sluggish.

But here is the good news: You can take proactive steps to keep your gut and brain in sync. Actions like maintaining a balanced diet, managing stress, and seeking professional help when needed can contribute to improved gut health, reducing symptoms of anxiety or depression and enhancing cognitive function. Embracing this holistic approach acknowledges the powerful gut–brain connection, helping you optimize your overall well-being.

Your gut is not just the headquarters of your digestion—it is a key player in your emotional and mental state. Understanding this link empowers you to take charge of your physical and mental health. So, let us next look at how gut health impacts your emotions and cognitive function.

YOUR GUT HEALTH

Your gut health is the master switch that controls all of the systems in your body. When things go awry in your digestive tract, you may experience a ripple effect on other bodily systems. For example, the health status of your gut influences your metabolism and immune system, as well as controlling the extraction of nutrients from your food and their absorption into the bloodstream. Consequently, taking care to maintain optimal gut health has knock-on benefits for the rest of your body.

Nutrient Absorption

The main function of your digestive tract is to extract nutrients from the food you eat so they can be absorbed into your bloodstream and taken to where they are needed to support your body's vast array of biological processes. As such, you can think of your gut as the gatekeeper that turns food into the essential nutrients your body requires. When your gut is not in its best shape, it can interfere with this crucial task. This means that your body might not get all of the vitamins, minerals, and other important nutrients necessary for it to function correctly (Hadadi et al., 2021), making it like a factory with some machines out of order.

Immune System and Inflammation

Your gut plays a vital role in your body's defenses and is staffed with a mighty army of immune cells. These cells are the protectors of your body, always on the lookout for troublemakers. When your gut is healthy, it supports these soldiers and enables them to do their work effectively and efficiently, keeping your body safe from infections and in perfect balance (Yoo et al., 2020).

Your gut and immune system are tight-knit buddies. A healthy digestive tract with a balanced colony of beneficial microorganisms helps to control the body's inflammatory response. On the other hand, an imbalance between good and bad microbes in the gut can trigger inflammation. This can lead to numerous problems throughout your body, from autoimmune diseases to heart problems, obesity, and even certain types of cancer (Vetrani et al., 2022). It is like a domino effect with your gut at the center.

Energy and Metabolism

The microorganisms living in your gut are not just hitchhikers—they have several essential functions that support human health. For one thing, they help with your energy and metabolism by breaking down tricky carbohydrates your body cannot digest itself and converting them into energy-packed molecules called short-chain fatty acids. These molecules keep your body going and help to control your metabolism (Martinez et al., 2016).

Skin Health

Your gut health can even affect your skin. Although skin disorders often have unique underlying causes, when your gut microbiota is out of balance, the resulting inflammation can weaken your gut's defenses, allowing large particles and toxins to pass through the gut lining into your bloodstream. This is commonly referred to as leaky gut and may show up on your skin as acne, eczema, and even psoriasis (Mahmud et al., 2022).

Consider your gut as the maestro of your body's orchestra. When it is in harmony, your body performs at its best. However, when things go off-key, it can affect every part of your health. Understanding this connection empowers you to take charge of your gut health and, in turn, your overall well-being.

Let us unravel more secrets about your gut and its incredible influence!

THE FANTASTIC WORLD OF YOUR GUT MICROBIOTA

The immense significance of the gut microbiota is a relatively new scientific discovery and our understanding continues to evolve rapidly. Scientists have not only discovered the trillions of microorganisms living within each of us but also begun to unravel their impact on the entire body. Instead of viewing them as parasitic hitchhikers, it is now understood that they are critical for human life, and we must engage in healthy lifestyle habits that support the well-being of these mysterious critters.

What Is the Gut Microbiota?

Inside your intestines lives a thriving community of microorganisms collectively referred to as the gut microbiota. This community consists of bacteria, viruses, fungi, and other microbes that have all set up shop in your gastrointestinal tract (Thursby & Juge, 2017). It is like a bustling town with different characters living together in harmony—ideally, at least! Let us explore why the gut microbiota matters.

The Gut Microbiota's Essential Role

Your gut microbiota is the unsung hero of your gut health. These microbes are not just along for a free ride—they work hard to keep your gut in tip-top shape. When your gut microbiota is in a healthy balance with an abundance of beneficial bacteria, it acts like a security guard, shielding your gut from harmful invaders and helping to prevent infection.

It also assists with digestion and nutrient absorption and even produces vital nutrients for your body, such as vitamin K and certain B vitamins. Moreover, it helps your body metabolize indigestible food components, producing energy for the gut lining as well as molecules that support your overall health.

In addition, the gut microbiota keeps your immune system on track by regulating the body's inflammatory response and training the all-important cells of your immune system to recognize harmful substances.

Thus, your gut microbiota is a natural multitasker! While it is busy digesting your food, synthesizing nutrients, and boosting your immune system, your gut microbiota communicates with your brain through the gut–brain connection. In this way, it affects your mood, emotions, and brain function.

8 Factors That Influence Your Gut Microbiota

Your gut microbiota is a flourishing colony of beneficial microorganisms. However, like a vibrant garden, it has to be tended to and nourished to maintain the flora. Here are eight key factors that may affect your "gut garden" (Hasan & Yang, 2019):

1. **Dietary diversity**: Just as the flowers in your garden need a steady supply of essential nutrients, so too do the microbes living in your gut. Moreover, because each species has its own specific requirements and preferences, eating the same things over and over can make your gut garden less diverse. To keep it thriving, you need to ensure that your diet includes a variety of whole foods, like fruits, vegetables, and whole grains.
2. **Fiber**: You must provide fuel in the form of fiber for your gut bacteria to grow and flourish. These food components are called prebiotics, and they serve as the water and sunlight for your gut garden. Prebiotics are found in foods such as fruits, vegetables, and whole grains and help your friendly gut bacteria thrive.
3. **Alcohol consumption**: Too much alcohol is like a tornado in your gut garden. It can harm the balance of your gut bacteria. However, moderate sipping of red wine, which contains potent antioxidants called polyphenols, can also help your gut bacteria stay healthy. As such, moderation is the key here.
4. **Antibiotics**: Antibiotics are like the security forces that come in to fight off infections, but they can be a bit too gung-ho. They not only knock out the bad guys but also disrupt the good bacteria in your gut. Even a single course of antibiotics can unsettle the delicate balance of your gut microbiota.

5. **Exercise**: The benefits of exercise for your body are well known, but did you know that it is also good for your gut? Studies show that physically active people have a more diverse gut community of friendly bacteria. If you are not that active, your gut might be missing out on some buddies.
6. **Tobacco smoking**: Smoking can cause problems in various parts of your body, and your gut is no exception. It affects the variety of bacteria in your gut and can increase the risk of conditions like inflammatory bowel disease. The good news? If you quit smoking, your gut can bounce back.
7. **Sleep**: Your gut loves a good bedtime routine. When you have an irregular sleep pattern, it can interfere with the microbial balance in your gut. So, if you want a happy gut, get your sleeping habits right.
8. **Chronic stress**: Persistently high stress levels can destroy some of your friendly gut bacteria, disrupting the balance between the good guys and the bad guys.

How to Tell When Your Gut Is Not Well

Because your gut health has far-reaching effects throughout your entire body, it is helpful to be able to recognize when things are not as they should be. Being mindful of your digestive system and the signs it gives out when it is calling for help allows you to take corrective action before the problem gets out of hand. Below you will find six telltale signs that your gut health is in trouble (NUHS Team, 2018):

1. **Unintentional weight changes**: If your weight suddenly goes up or down without you changing your eating or workout habits, it could indicate a problem with your gut health that is interfering with how your body absorbs nutrients and stores fat.
2. **Skin irritation**: Skin problems such as eczema and psoriasis may be linked to your gut's bacterial buddies. Lower levels of good microorganisms can affect your immune system and increase inflammation, which may make itself known on your skin.
3. **Upset stomach**: A perfectly healthy digestive system breaks down your food, absorbs nutrients, and eliminates waste products smoothly and efficiently. When your gut health is compromised, you may start to notice symptoms like diarrhea, constipation, bloating, and abdominal pain.
4. **Sleep disturbances and constant fatigue**: Since your gut health is linked to the balance of chemicals in your brain, changes to your gut microbiota can affect your sleep. If you find it difficult to get to sleep, have a hard time sleeping throughout the night, or wake up feeling tired the next day, it may be related to poor gut health. An imbalance in your gut microbiota can also cause general fatigue due to changes in your metabolism.
5. **Autoimmune conditions**: An unhealthy gut often takes its toll on the immune system. Higher levels of inflammation and an immune system that overreacts to perceived threats may eventually turn on your own cells and tissues, resulting in autoimmune conditions such as thyroid problems, multiple sclerosis, and rheumatoid arthritis.
6. **Food intolerance**: Intolerance to certain foods may be caused by several factors related to poor digestion and an unhealthy gut. For example, lactose intolerance originates from low levels of the enzyme lactase, which is normally

responsible for breaking down this sugar. If your gut is unhealthy, the amount of lactase produced in your small intestine can drop, meaning that the lactose instead gets fermented by the gut bacteria, causing bloating, pain, and an urgent need to go to the toilet.

COMMON GUT ISSUES UNRAVELED

Gut health can be challenging. Sometimes, you are completely unaware of the problem and may have some minor symptoms like occasional bloating. However, the more severe the problem becomes, the more it feels like your digestive system is throwing a little tantrum. You start noticing more debilitating symptoms throughout your gut. Some of the more common digestive problems caused by poor gut health are outlined below (Singh et al., 2021).

Irritable Bowel Syndrome (IBS)

IBS is a common gut disorder with symptoms that include abdominal pain, bloating, and changes in bowel habits such as diarrhea, constipation, or a combination of both. Unlike inflammatory bowel diseases such as Crohn's disease and ulcerative colitis (see below), IBS does not cause inflammation or permanent damage to the digestive tract. Nonetheless, its chronic nature can significantly impact a person's quality of life.

Celiac Disease

Imagine your body being on high alert when it encounters gluten. That is what happens with celiac disease, an autoimmune disorder where gluten is the enemy. When gluten enters the scene, it triggers a battle in your small intestine, causing damage and digestive problems. If you have celiac disease, you may experience digestive issues like abdominal pain, diarrhea, and unwanted weight loss.

Chronic Diarrhea

The occasional bout of diarrhea is fairly common, but when it sticks around for more than a few days, it becomes a problem. Chronic diarrhea can have many causes, including infections, digestive disorders, medication, or underlying health issues. If left unchecked, it can lead to dehydration and nutrient deficiencies.

Constipation

Constipation is like an unwanted guest overstaying its welcome. It happens when you have infrequent trips to the bathroom or struggle to pass stool. Low-fiber diets, not drinking enough water, being a couch potato, certain medications, or underlying health problems are among the common culprits.

Gastroesophageal Reflux Disease (GERD)

Picture your stomach acid having a little party in your esophagus. That is what GERD does. It is a chronic condition where stomach acid splashes back into the esophagus, causing symptoms like heartburn, regurgitation, chest pain, and swallowing difficulties. If left untreated, it can lead to more severe issues.

Peptic Ulcer Disease

Peptic ulcers are like little sores in your stomach or upper small intestine. They are often caused by a bacterium called *Helicobacter pylori* or the overuse of certain pain medications, such as nonsteroidal anti-inflammatory drugs. These ulcers can cause stomach pain, bloating, nausea, and sometimes bleeding.

Crohn's Disease

Crohn's disease is an inflammatory bowel condition primarily targeting your digestive tract. It causes inflammation and damage to your intestines, leading to symptoms like abdominal pain, diarrhea, weight loss, fatigue, and malnutrition.

Ulcerative Colitis

Ulcerative colitis is another inflammatory bowel disease marked by chronic inflammation and ulcers in your colon and rectum. Symptoms can include abdominal pain, bloody diarrhea, rectal bleeding, fatigue, and unwanted weight loss.

Gallstones

Gallstones are like tiny pebbles that form in your gallbladder, often made of cholesterol. They can block your bile ducts, leading to upper abdominal pain, nausea, vomiting, and jaundice (yellowish skin and eyes).

Pancreatitis

Pancreatitis is a painful condition resulting from an inflamed pancreas. It can be a quick hit (acute) or a long-term annoyance (chronic). Acute pancreatitis is often caused by gallstones or excessive alcohol consumption, leading to severe abdominal pain, nausea, and vomiting. Chronic pancreatitis is a persistent issue, involving ongoing inflammation and permanent pancreas damage.

Liver Disease

Your liver is a superstar among your body's organs, but it can also get sick. Common liver problems include hepatitis, cirrhosis, and fatty liver disease. A sick liver can show up as jaundice, constant fatigue, abdominal pain, swelling due to water retention, and changes to your appetite and weight.

Diverticulitis

Diverticulitis occurs when little pouches (diverticula) form in your colon. These pouches can sometimes become inflamed or infected, leading to symptoms such as abdominal pain, fever, nausea, and changes in your bathroom habits.

Food Intolerance

Have you ever had trouble digesting certain foods? If so, your body may be deficient in some key enzymes, making it hard to break down specific foods. The most common culprits are lactose (a sugar found in dairy products) and gluten (a protein found in wheat, barley, and rye). When this happens, you might get bloated, feel gassy, or have stomach pain. However, do not worry—it is not life-threatening. You can manage food intolerance by avoiding or limiting your consumption of the corresponding foods or using enzyme supplements to aid digestion.

Food Allergies

Food allergies are somewhat more straightforward because they lead to immediate reactions like hives, swelling, and even difficulty breathing. Special tests and elimination diets can help pinpoint the foods causing these problems.

Food Sensitivities

Food sensitivities, also known as non-IgE-mediated food allergies, are where your digestive system does not react well to certain foods. Unlike regular allergies, these sensitivities can take hours or even days to develop. Figuring them out can be tricky, but by eliminating potentially problematic food items and reintroducing them one at a time, you can identify any foods that are troublesome for you.

Overall, gut issues can be extremely difficult to diagnose, and unfortunately many people suffer for years before finally stumbling upon an answer. Rest assured that there is a reason for your grumbly tummy! If you have undergone all of the tests and investigations only to come up empty-handed, the problem may lie within your gut microbiota. The good news is that there are actions you can take that are straightforward and within your control.

In the next chapter, we will dive into our first hack—the importance of hydration for maintaining a healthy gut and overall wellness. It is all about keeping it simple and affordable by drinking enough water for improved gut health. Stay tuned!

2

HACK #1: BOTTOMS UP

HYDRATE YOUR WAY TO A HAPPY GUT

> *"Drinking water is like washing out your insides. The water will cleanse the system, fill you up, decrease your caloric load, and improve the function of all your tissues."*
>
> — KEVIN R. STONE, MD, THE STONE CLINIC, USA

Water, the elixir of life, is an essential component for maintaining overall health and well-being. However, the impact of proper hydration on gut health is often overlooked. Drinking water is one of the easiest and cheapest ways to improve gut health, yet many people skip this simple habit. This chapter aims to shed light on the significance of water in promoting a healthy gut and explores the reasons why it is so common to neglect this fundamental practice.

HYDRATION AND GUT HEALTH

Drinking enough water helps your digestive system work smoothly (Popkin et al., 2010). It assists in breaking down your food, makes digestion easier, and improves nutrient absorption. Staying hydrated also helps to keep your stools soft and regular, preventing uncomfortable constipation. Furthermore, sufficient hydration plays an essential role in maintaining a good balance of friendly bacteria in your gut, which, as we have learned, is crucial for digestion and overall well-being. Giving your body enough water creates an ideal environment for these beneficial microorganisms to thrive. That means a healthier gut microbiota and better digestive health for you!

It can be an eye-opener for any individual to see how a simple thing like hydration can positively impact their gut health. People who suffer from digestive issues like bloating and irregular bowel movements who make a conscious effort to drink more water throughout the day can significantly improve their gut health over time. Keeping yourself hydrated is a straightforward way to support your gut and maintain your digestion in tip-top shape!

You may ask how the basic act of drinking water can make such a difference to your digestive system. Let us find out.

How Hydration Affects Your Digestive System

Sufficient saliva: When you are hydrated, your body can make more saliva, which helps break down your food right from the start of chewing. Saliva contains an enzyme called amylase that helps digest carbohydrates, like those present in bread, pasta, and potatoes, for example.

Digestion: Water plays a crucial supporting role for the digestive enzymes in your intestines that break down food. These little workers split the chemical bonds in proteins, fats, and carbohydrates to release the nutrients your body needs. However, they must be able to access them first. If not enough water is present, the enzymes cannot come into adequate contact with the food particles and their chemical bonds to break them down effectively.

Nutrient transport: Water is like an efficient vehicle that transports nutrients to where they are needed. Think of your intestines as a riverbed. When there is a drought and the riverbed has dried up, nothing can be carried downstream. However, when it rains regularly, the water level rises and the river flows, carrying sand and sticks downstream with it. Similarly, when there is enough water in your digestive tract, it mixes with the food you eat, giving it a more fluid consistency and making it easier to pass through the intestines. Water is also essential for transporting nutrients across the gut lining. This process can be compared to the absorption of water by the soil next to the river, which allows plants to grow on the riverbank.

Smooth moves: After assisting with digestion, water helps your body get rid of waste. When you are dehydrated, your body tries to retain as much water as possible, making your stool hard and difficult to pass as the contents of your colon become dry. Drinking enough water, however, helps keep food and waste products moving smoothly through your intestines and ensures that your stool does not get stuck.

Let us next consider six further reasons why drinking water is not only a good idea to help your digestive system but also essential for your gut health.

6 Reasons Hydration Is Essential for Gut Health

1. **Improved digestion and nutrient absorption**: Water adds fluid to the contents of your intestines, making it easier for

the food to move through the gut and get broken down and for the nutrients to be absorbed.
2. **Better bowel regularity**: When the body is dehydrated, the colon absorbs more water from the waste, which leads to dry and hard stools that are difficult to pass. Maintaining adequate hydration thus helps prevent the common problem of constipation.
3. **Enhanced gut motility**: Hydration supports proper gut motility—the movement of food through the digestive system. Being well hydrated also supports the natural contractions of the intestines, known as peristalsis, that help move food along. Healthy gut motility prevents issues like bloating, gas, and abdominal discomfort.
4. **More balanced gut microbiota**: Not drinking enough water can disrupt the balance of the gut microorganisms, leading to dysbiosis and associated digestive problems. Adequate hydration helps create a favorable environment for the gut microbiota, allowing it to thrive and carry out its vital functions.
5. **Reduced gut inflammation**: Inflammation in the digestive tract causes discomfort and can interfere with the normal functioning of the gut. Drinking enough water helps keep the gut lining moist, providing a protective barrier against irritation from the intestinal contents. By reducing gut inflammation, you help promote a healthier digestive system and support your immune system.
6. **Lower risk of a leaky gut**: A leaky gut develops when the lining of the digestive tract becomes more porous, allowing larger molecules to pass through into the bloodstream. Even mild dehydration over a prolonged period can contribute to this condition, which may cause a range of symptoms from skin rashes to anxiety and persistent gut issues such as bloating, constipation, or

diarrhea. Maintaining proper hydration supports the natural structure and function of the gut lining and reduces the risk of developing a leaky gut and resulting health issues.

What Are the Effects of Dehydration on Gut Health?

Dehydration can have numerous adverse effects on your digestive system, as outlined below (El-Sharkawy et al., 2015).

Sluggish digestion: When you do not drink enough water, your digestive system does not work as smoothly as it should. This slows down the processes of breaking down the food you eat and absorbing the essential nutrients your body needs. Digestive issues like gas, bloating, and constipation may occur, as well as nutrient deficiencies.

Stomach ulcers: Not drinking sufficient water can increase your chance of developing stomach ulcers, which are painful sores in your stomach lining. Dehydration also makes it easier for harmful bacteria to grow in your gut, leading to infections and other digestive issues.

Irritated insides: When you are dehydrated, your gut can become inflamed and irritated. This may contribute to conditions like IBS, where your tummy feels upset much of the time. It can also weaken the gut lining, increasing your risk of developing a leaky gut.

Detoxification difficulties: Your colon needs water to eliminate waste and toxins. Dehydration may mean that your body has a hard time flushing out these harmful substances, which puts extra stress on your liver and other organs responsible for detoxification. Over time, this can affect how well your gut functions and how efficiently it removes waste from your body.

However, dehydration does not only affect your digestive system. Water is critical for the structure and function of all parts of your body, and so not drinking enough can cause a wide range of additional symptoms (El-Sharkawy et al., 2015):

Brain fog and headaches: When you are dehydrated, your brain cannot function at its best. You may experience difficulty concentrating, poor memory, and decreased mental clarity. This can make you feel foggy or "out of it." Dehydration can also trigger headaches or worsen existing ones, leaving you feeling uncomfortable and unable to focus.

Dry and flaky skin: Your skin is the largest and most exposed organ in your body, and it needs proper hydration to stay healthy. If you are dehydrated, your skin may become dry, flaky, and lacking in elasticity. It can also lose its natural glow and appear dull. Proper hydration helps moisturize your skin and contributes to a more vibrant and youthful appearance.

Muscle weakness and fatigue: Water is essential for maintaining muscle function. It is crucial for the movements of minerals such as sodium, magnesium, and calcium needed for muscle tissues to contract. Therefore, when you are dehydrated, your muscles may not have sufficient water either, leading to weakness and fatigue. This can affect your physical performance, making it more difficult to exercise or engage in other activities.

Weight loss difficulties: Water plays a vital role in the breakdown and utilization of fat, so staying hydrated is crucial when trying to lose weight. Dehydration can also often be mistaken for hunger, leading to unnecessary snacking or overeating. Moreover, when you are dehydrated, your metabolism may slow down, making it harder to shed those extra pounds.

In a nutshell, not drinking enough water can harm your gut health as well as your overall well-being. It can slow digestion, cause constipation, increase your risk of digestive issues, induce inflammation and irritation in your gut, and impair your body's natural detoxification processes. In order to keep your gut healthy, it is imperative to drink sufficient water throughout the day and listen to your body's thirst signals. By staying hydrated, you will be supporting the health of your gut and entire body.

HOW MUCH WATER SHOULD YOU BE DRINKING?

Factors Affecting Recommended Water Intake

The amount of water you need depends on a few things, but to keep it simple, adults should generally aim to drink about 8 cups (approximately 2 liters or 64 ounces) of water daily. However, everyone is different and your exact requirements will also vary with factors such as your age, activity level, and environment (Harvard T.H. Chan School of Public Health, n.d.):

Age: Children and teenagers do not need as much water as adults. Children up to the age of 8 should consume 4 to 5 cups per day (0.9–1.2 liters or 32–40 ounces), tweens need about 7 to 8 cups (1.7–1.9 liters or 56–64 ounces), and teenagers typically require 8 to 11 cups (1.9–2.6 liters or 64–88 ounces).

Men vs. women: Men typically need more water than women. They tend to have more lean muscle mass, and as we learned above muscles require water to work well. The recommended daily water intake is 13 cups (3.1 liters or 104 ounces) for adult men and 9 cups (2.1 liters or 72 ounces) for adult women, although pregnant or breastfeeding women may require up to 10 to 13 cups (2.4–3.1 liters or 80–104 ounces). Remember, this includes all fluids from hot and cold beverages as well as food, not just plain water.

Activity level: When you are physically active, such as playing sports or doing exercise, your body sweats and loses water. This means you need to drink more water to stay hydrated. Before exercising, drink a cup or two of water, and during exercise, have a few sips every 15 minutes. Afterward, drink more water to rehydrate.

Hot environment: If you live in a warmer climate, you will need to consume more water to replace that lost through sweating.

How to Estimate Your Water Needs

Do not worry—you do not need to be a math genius. Here is a simple way to figure out how much water you should drink based on your weight (Ahmad, 2015):

For every pound (about half a kilogram) you weigh, try to drink half an ounce to one ounce of water each day. For example, if you weigh 150 pounds (68 kilograms), you should aim to drink around 75 to 150 ounces (2.2 to 4.4 liters) of water daily.

10 Simple Rules to Stay Hydrated

Here are some easy-to-remember tips to ensure you are getting enough water:

1. **Drink before you are thirsty**: Thirst is your body's way of saying it needs water. However, do not wait until you are parched. Sip water throughout the day, even if you do not feel thirsty. For example, you could set an alarm on your phone reminding you to drink a glass of water every hour while at work. This will maintain your hydration levels and make you feel more refreshed.

2. **Drink before exercise**: If you are going to play sports or do any activities that make you sweat, drink water before you begin. This will help you stay hydrated and perform better.
3. **Check your urine**: Yes, you read it right. Take a peek at your urine. If it is light yellow or clear, that means you are drinking enough water. If it is darker, it is a sign that you need to drink more.
4. **Drink water when you wake up and before bed**: Start and end your day with a glass of water. This provides a simple way to kickstart hydration in the morning and rehydrate before sleep.
5. **Set a daily goal**: Decide on a specific amount of water you want to drink daily, such as a certain number of cups or bottles. Setting goals like this can help you stay on track.
6. **Keep a reusable water bottle with you wherever you go**: By doing this, you will always have water within reach and can sip on it throughout the day.
7. **Replace sugary drinks with water**: Instead of reaching for sodas, juices, or other sugary beverages, try replacing them with water. Water is a healthier option and can quench your thirst just as well, maybe even better.
8. **Drink water before meals**: Have a glass of water prior to each meal. This helps you stay hydrated and may even make you eat less, which is good for your overall health.
9. **Add flavor to your water**: If you find plain water too boring, feel free to experiment by adding slices of fruit like lemon or cucumber to give it a refreshing taste. You can also try sugar-free water flavorings. If you are concerned about the quality of your tap water, think about investing in a water filter, which can remove impurities and make your water taste better.

10. **Eat water-rich foods**: Include fruits and vegetables such as watermelons, oranges, cucumbers, and strawberries in your diet. The high water content of these foods can contribute to your overall hydration.

These tips are just suggestions, and listening to your own body's signals is essential. Basically, if you feel thirsty, drink water. Stay mindful of your hydration needs, and make the conscious decision to drink more water throughout the day. Remember, water is your body's best friend, and it helps you stay energized, focused, and healthy. So, make it a habit to drink enough water every day.

WATER-RICH FOODS FOR HYDRATION

Water-rich foods can be your secret weapon if you are looking for tasty ways to stay hydrated. The high water content of these foods can help quench your thirst and keep you hydrated throughout the day (Popkin et al., 2010).

Here are some examples of water-rich foods:

- **Watermelons**: Watermelons are about 92% water, making them a perfect hydrating snack on a hot summer day.
- **Cucumbers**: Besides being cool and refreshing, cucumbers contain approximately 96% water. They add a delightful crunch while keeping you hydrated.
- **Strawberries**: Berries are delicious and contain about 91% water. You can enjoy them as a snack or in a smoothie, or even add them to your morning cereal.
- **Oranges**: Oranges are bursting with flavor and contain around 87% water. They are an excellent choice for a hydrating citrusy treat.

- **Pineapples**: With a water content of about 87%, pineapples are delicious and contribute to your hydration levels.
- **Lettuce**: Lettuce varieties like romaine or iceberg are over 90% water, making them a hydrating choice for your salads and sandwiches.
- **Tomatoes**: Tomatoes are about 94% water, making them a refreshing addition to your salads and sandwiches. They can even be enjoyed as a snack.
- **Bell peppers**: Picture a vibrant plate of colorful bell peppers—red, green, and yellow. These crunchy vegetables contain around 92% water, adding hydration and a pleasing crunch to your meals.
- **Grapes**: These bite-sized fruits are not only delicious but also contain about 81% water. They make for a refreshing snack that will also satisfy your thirst.
- **Celery**: With a water content of approximately 95%, celery is a hydrating vegetable that can add a satisfying crunch to your snacks.
- **Spinach**: Help your body hydrate by preparing a bowl of fresh, leafy spinach. It can be enjoyed in a salad or sautéed in a stir-fry. Spinach is about 91% water, making it a nutritious and hydrating choice for your meals.
- **Coconut water**: Coconut water is delicious and a natural source of hydration, containing electrolytes that help replenish your body's fluids.
- **Broccoli**: This cruciferous vegetable comprises about 89% water, providing hydration as well as valuable nutrients.
- **Peaches**: Peaches contain about 89% water and can be a hydrating and delightful fruit to enjoy during the summer.

Incorporating water-rich foods into your daily routine in the form of various fruits and vegetables can contribute to your overall hydration and well-being. So, the next time you are looking for a tasty and hydrating snack, reach for these water-packed options to quench your thirst and nourish your body.

ARE ALL BEVERAGES CREATED EQUAL?

Not all drinks offer the same benefits for hydration. It is important to know which drinks to choose and how to balance them to stay properly hydrated. When it comes to hydrating your body, nothing beats good old water. It is the best choice because your body can easily absorb it to replenish fluids lost through sweating and other bodily functions. So, make sure to drink plenty of plain water throughout the day.

Sports drinks can be helpful if you take part in intense physical activity like working out. They are designed to replace electrolytes and fluids lost during exercise. Electrolytes are charged minerals such as sodium and potassium that your body needs for many of its functions, such as muscle contractions and nerve transmission. Sports drinks usually also contain carbohydrates. As a result, they help restore your body's electrolyte balance and give you some energy (Shirreffs, 2009).

Some fruit juices, like watermelon juice or coconut water, also contain high levels of electrolytes and help to hydrate you. Their high water content can help quench your thirst, especially when it is hot outside. Just keep in mind that most fruit juices are high in sugar and low in fiber, so do not overdo it (Gutierrez et al., 2022).

Now, let us talk about drinks that may have the opposite effect and dehydrate you. First, the caffeine in beverages such as coffee and tea can have a diuretic effect. This means that it makes you produce more urine, which can lead to greater fluid loss. However, the diuretic effect of caffeine is usually mild, unless you drink a lot of it or are particularly sensitive (Seal et al., 2017).

Second, alcoholic drinks are also diuretic. When you drink alcohol, it stops your body from releasing a hormone called vasopressin that helps you retain water. This can make you pee more and leave you dehydrated. So, if you are drinking alcohol, make sure to consume water or other non-alcoholic drinks alongside it to stay hydrated (Polhuis et al., 2017).

Finally, sodas and some flavored drinks may not be diuretic on their own but can make you dehydrated if you drink too much. They are often high in sugar and caffeine, which can increase urination and exert a diuretic effect (Dibay Moghadam et al., 2020).

What does the science say about different beverages and their effects on your hydration status?

Plain water: Many athletes and healthcare professionals emphasize the importance of staying hydrated with water during physical activities or in hot weather. For instance, the American College of Sports Medicine recommends drinking water before, during, and after exercise to maintain proper hydration levels (Convertino et al., 1996).

Sports drinks: Researchers have examined the effectiveness of sports drinks in aiding hydration during exercise. For example, studies have indicated that consuming a sports drink containing carbohydrates and electrolytes helps maintain hydration and improve endurance during prolonged exercise compared with the consumption of water alone (von Duvillard et al., 2004).

Caffeinated beverages: Research suggests that caffeinated beverages like coffee and tea, while mildly diuretic, still contribute to overall fluid balance. A study published in *PLOS ONE* reported that moderate caffeine consumption (approximately four cups of coffee per day) did not significantly impact hydration status, indicating that caffeine-containing drinks still count toward a person's total daily fluid intake (Killer et al., 2014).

Alcohol: As many of us may know, drinking large amounts of alcohol can lead to a hangover (Koob, 2019). One of the reasons you may feel queasy or suffer from a headache after a night of drinking is that alcohol suppresses the release of the hormone vasopressin, which tells your kidneys to retain water. Consequently, you probably go to the toilet more when you have a lot to drink, resulting in dehydration. Some people find that by alternating alcoholic beverages with water or other non-alcoholic drinks, they can avoid the dehydration associated with drinking alcohol.

In short, these examples highlight how different beverages can have varying impacts on your hydration levels. While water remains the optimal choice for hydration, sports drinks may be beneficial during intense physical activity. Caffeinated beverages can also contribute to overall hydration, but it is important to limit consumption. By contrast, alcoholic drinks can lead to dehydration if consumed in excess and not balanced with sufficient water intake. By understanding these basics, you can make smart choices to stay hydrated and keep your body healthy.

The next chapter will focus on how fiber promotes our digestive health, supports regular bowel movements, and nourishes beneficial gut bacteria. It will provide practical tips for incorporating more fiber into your diet, helping you improve your gut health through wise dietary choices.

HACK #2: BOOST YOUR GUT HEALTH WITH FIBER

THE IMPORTANCE OF FIBER

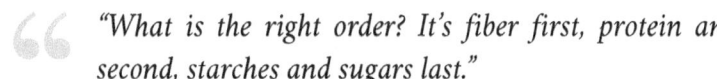
"What is the right order? It's fiber first, protein and fat second, starches and sugars last."

— JESSIE INCHAUSPÉ, GLUCOSE REVOLUTION

In today's fast-paced world, processed foods have become a significant part of our diet. Despite their convenience, these foods are often low in fiber and high in unhealthy fats and additives.

Unfortunately, most people in Europe and North America consume less fiber than recommended, which is partially attributable to the increasing consumption of processed and fast foods high in sugar, fat, and animal protein. According to an article published on the UCSF Health website entitled "Increasing Fiber Intake," the American Heart Association Eating Plan recommends consuming 25–30 grams of dietary fiber from food sources daily. However, the article highlights that many adults in the

United States fall short of this recommendation, with an average intake of only 15 grams per day, roughly half of the recommended amount (UCSF Health, n.d.).

Fiber comes from plants and is an essential component of our diet. It is composed of complex structures that our bodies cannot fully break down, such as the walls of plant cells. While many people associate fiber with promoting regular bowel movements, it actually plays a much more significant role in our overall health, especially in terms of supporting beneficial gut bacteria.

In this chapter, we will focus on the benefits of fiber for gut health and learn some valuable tips for increasing our fiber intake. Transitioning from a diet centered around processed foods to one that emphasizes fiber intake can be overwhelming for many people. Therefore, we should first explore exactly why fiber is so important for the gastrointestinal system before looking at some practical suggestions for incorporating more fiber-rich foods into our daily meals.

FIBER AND GUT HEALTH

What Is Fiber?

Fiber is the champion of your gut health. It mostly consists of the tough parts of plant cells that give them structure and support. Examples of high-fiber foods include whole grains like oatmeal and brown rice, fruits such as apples and berries, vegetables like broccoli and carrots, and legumes such as beans, lentils, and chickpeas. When you eat fiber, it passes through your digestive system mostly unchanged until it reaches your colon and its flourishing population of gut microorganisms. These trillions of tiny helpers do what our own bodies could not, happily munching on the fiber and breaking it down into helpful substances such as short-chain fatty acids. These substances provide nourishment to the cells lining your colon, promote a healthy gut environment, and support your immune system. It is like throwing a big feast for our gut microbiota to keep it happy and thriving (Barber et al., 2020).

Benefits of a High-Fiber Diet

Eating a diet rich in fiber has several important benefits:

Fiber helps normalize bowel movements: One of the most crucial functions of fiber is adding bulk to your stool, making it easier for you to have regular bowel movements. Without enough fiber, things can get "backed up" and you may experience constipation. Here is a simple analogy to explain the importance of fiber: Imagine you have a sink drain that gradually gets clogged up with food particles and gunk. Without a drain cleaner, the water does not flow properly and you end up with a big mess. Fiber is like the drain cleaner for your gut—it keeps everything moving smoothly, prevents clogs, and ensures a healthy gut environment.

Fiber helps maintain bowel health: Fiber also nourishes the good microbes living in your gut, paying them back for the critical role they play in keeping you healthy. When they feast on fiber, they produce beneficial compounds that help reduce inflammation and support a strong immune system. Think of fiber as their favorite meal; when they are happy, you are happy too!

Fiber lowers cholesterol levels: Some types of fiber, particularly soluble fiber found in foods like oats, fruit, and beans, bind to cholesterol in your digestive system. This helps remove cholesterol from your body, reducing the levels of "bad" low-density lipoprotein (LDL) cholesterol in your blood. This assists with keeping your arteries clean and can reduce your risk of heart disease.

Fiber helps control blood sugar: Fiber, especially soluble fiber, slows down the absorption of sugar into your bloodstream after a meal. This helps regulate your blood sugar levels, which is particularly beneficial if you suffer from diabetes. In this way, fiber acts like a traffic cop regulating the flow of sugar in your body, preventing spikes and crashes.

Fiber aids in achieving a healthy weight: High-fiber foods are often more filling and lower in calories. Eating them provides a sense of fullness and satisfaction, reducing your likelihood of overeating and helping you maintain a healthy weight.

Fiber helps you live longer: Research suggests that people who consume a high-fiber diet tend to have a lower risk of chronic diseases such as heart disease, strokes, type 2 diabetes, and certain kinds of cancer.

HOW MUCH FIBER SHOULD YOU BE EATING?

The suggested daily fiber intakes for different age groups and genders are as follows, based on recommendations from the U.S. Department of Agriculture's *Dietary Guidelines for Americans* (McKeown et al., 2022):

- Women under 50: 25–28 grams of fiber per day.
- Men under 50: 31–34 grams of fiber per day.
- Women 51 and older: 22 grams of fiber per day.
- Men 51 and older: 28 grams of fiber per day.
- Children: The recommended intake varies with age. As a general rule, children older than one year should aim for their age in grams plus 5 grams. For example, a 5-year-old child should consume approximately 10 grams of fiber per day (5 + 5 grams).

Below are some examples of fiber-rich foods and their approximate fiber contents to help you meet your daily fiber goals. These values were taken from the Mayo Clinic website (Mayo Clinic, 2023).

- 1 medium-sized apple (with skin): 4.5 grams
- 1 cup of cooked oatmeal: 4.0 grams
- 1 cup of cooked brown rice: 3.5 grams
- 1 cup of cooked black beans: 15.0 grams
- 1 slice of whole wheat bread: 2.0 grams

To reach your daily fiber intake, it is a good idea to include a variety of fiber-rich foods in your meals and snacks throughout the day. It is also better to eat more whole foods that have been minimally processed and thus still contain most of their fiber. For example, you could choose whole grain bread instead of white bread, brown rice instead of white rice, and whole wheat pasta instead of regular pasta.

It is best to gradually increase your fiber intake, as fiber is a type of carbohydrate. Make sure to drink plenty of water to help the fiber move smoothly through your digestive system. To summarize, aim for your recommended daily fiber intake based on your age and gender, and keep your gut happy and healthy!

TYPES OF FIBER: SOLUBLE VS. INSOLUBLE

There are two main types of fiber: insoluble fiber, also known as roughage, and soluble fiber. Neither of them can be digested by the human digestive system, and each type has different functions in the gut (Lattimer & Haub, 2010).

Soluble Fiber

Soluble fiber absorbs water and has a dense, slimy texture. It offers several health benefits, including the following:

- **Blood sugar control**: Soluble fiber slows down the absorption of sugars and stabilizes blood glucose levels, making it beneficial for people with insulin resistance, prediabetes, and type 2 diabetes.
- **Cholesterol management**: Soluble fiber traps cholesterol from food, preventing its absorption and helping lower LDL cholesterol levels in the blood, reducing the risk of heart disease.
- **Bile acid regulation**: Soluble fiber also traps bile acids, promoting their removal from the body. Because your body synthesizes these bile acids from cholesterol to aid in digestion, this forces your liver to make more and thereby also decreases blood cholesterol levels.
- **Satiety and weight loss**: Soluble fiber increases your feeling of fullness and delays hunger, contributing to weight loss and improved body mass index.
- **Gut microbiota support**: Soluble fiber acts as a prebiotic, undergoing fermentation by the beneficial bacteria in your gut to produce essential short-chain fatty acids.

Insoluble Fiber

Insoluble fiber is resistant to digestion and remains intact as it passes through the gastrointestinal tract. Its benefits include the following:

- **Relieving constipation**: Insoluble fiber adds bulk to your stool, absorbs water, and promotes regular bowel movements.
- **Promoting gut health**: While your gut microbiota has a minimal effect on insoluble fiber, it can help stimulate slow fermentation in the colon.

THE RISKS AND SIGNS OF TOO MUCH FIBER

Fiber is an essential dietary component that aids digestion and keeps you feeling full. However, just like everything in life, striking a balance is essential and consuming too much fiber can have certain downsides. Let us explore the risks and signs that there is too much fiber in your diet (Borkoles et al., 2022).

Abdominal Pain

Consuming too much fiber can lead to stomach pain and cramps, especially if you are not used to it. If your body is accustomed to foods low in fiber, even a tiny portion of fiber-rich food, such as bran flakes, may cause abdominal pain.

Mineral Deficiencies

Excessive consumption of fiber (especially from foods like bran and whole grains) can hinder your body's ability to absorb essential minerals such as iron, calcium, zinc, and magnesium. Thus, a fiber overdose prevents your body from getting the minerals it needs, leading to you feeling tired or weak or developing brittle nails. Remember, these risks are uncommon—most people can handle moderate to high amounts of fiber without any issues. However, if you notice any of these signs, listening to your body and adjusting your fiber intake is essential.

MY TIPS FOR INCORPORATING MORE FIBER INTO YOUR DIET

One key lesson I have learned is the importance of whole-food carbohydrate sources. By opting for whole fruits such as apples, oranges, or bananas instead of fruit juice, for example, you can enjoy the benefits of fiber while relishing the natural sweetness and nutritional goodness of tasty fruit. Additionally, leaving the skin on fruits and vegetables such as apples, cucumbers, and sweet potatoes adds an extra fiber punch to your meals, enhancing both taste and health benefits.

Another approach that has worked wonders for me is prioritizing vegetables in meals. By incorporating a generous portion of vegetables and making them the hero of the dish rather than a mere sidekick, I not only increase my fiber intake but also infuse my dishes with vibrant colors, textures, and flavors. Eating my vegetables first during meals ensures that I consume a substantial amount before moving on to other components.

As a fan of snacking, I have discovered the delightful world of popcorn. This is not only a satisfying and crunchy treat but also a fiber-rich snack option. By swapping processed snacks for a bowl of air-popped popcorn, I have found a guilt-free way to curb my cravings while boosting my daily fiber intake.

When it comes to sweet treats, have you heard of chia seeds? These tiny powerhouses of nutrition are packed with fiber, and incorporating them into my diet has made it easier for me to meet my body's fiber needs. From creating indulgent chia seed puddings to adding them to smoothies and baked goods, these versatile seeds offer a delightful and fiber-filled twist to my favorite recipes.

Furthermore, I have come to appreciate the beauty of whole fruits and vegetables rather than relying on their juice counterparts. By enjoying whole apples, pears, and other fruits, I savor the fiber-rich goodness and reap the benefits of their natural fiber. This provides me with a simple yet effective way to both enhance my diet and nourish my gut.

In my quest for healthy fats and fiber, avocados have become a cherished addition to my meals. Whether spread on whole grain toast or incorporated into salads, their creamy texture and fiber content make for a satisfying and nutritious choice.

I have also turned to nuts and seeds to keep my snacking options interesting. These nutrient-dense powerhouses provide a satisfying crunch and deliver a healthy dose of fiber. Whether enjoyed as a snack on their own or added to recipes such as salads, stir-fries, or granola bars, nuts and seeds have become a reliable source of fiber in my daily routine.

When baking, I have found that high-fiber flour, such as whole wheat or oat flour, adds depth and nutrition to my kitchen creations. From bread and muffins to cookies and pancakes, these alternative flours have provided me with a tasty way to incorporate more fiber into my baked goods.

The vibrant world of berries has also become a staple in my quest for fiber. Whether I add a handful of fresh or frozen blueberries, raspberries, or strawberries to my morning cereal or blend them into smoothies, berries bring a burst of flavor and fiber to my meals.

Moreover, I have discovered the immense benefits of legumes. From lentils and beans to chickpeas, incorporating these protein-rich powerhouses into my diet not only adds variety but also amps up the fiber content of my meals, especially in terms of soluble fiber. Whether preparing a hearty lentil soup or a zesty bean salad, legumes have become essential to my fiber-rich journey.

I have also learned the importance of mindful label reading. Taking the time to check food labels allows me to identify products rich in fiber. For a food to be considered high in fiber, it must contain at least 6 grams of fiber per 100 grams of food. By choosing foods with substantial fiber contents listed on their labels, I can make informed decisions that align with my goal of increasing fiber intake.

In my pursuit of optimal gut health, I strive to incorporate high-fiber foods into every meal. Whether I add a handful of spinach or kale to my morning smoothie, enjoy a side of steamed broccoli or green beans with dinner, or include fiber-rich grains like quinoa or bulgur in my lunchtime grain bowls, I aim to create well-rounded and fiber-packed meals throughout the day.

I have come to greatly appreciate the impact of fiber on my overall well-being and have witnessed firsthand the positive effects of incorporating more fiber into my diet. I am excited to share these insights with others on their own journeys toward a healthier gut and improved overall health—and that includes you.

In summary, these 11 simple tips can help you incorporate more fiber into your diet:

1. Choose whole fruit over fruit juice.
2. Do not peel your fruit and vegetables unless the skin is thick and inedible, as in the case of pumpkins.
3. Include vegetables with every meal and eat them first.
4. Eat popcorn as a snack in place of potato chips.
5. Snack on fruit.
6. Choose whole grains over refined grains.
7. Include chia seeds in your diet.
8. Nuts and seeds make for tasty, fiber-filled snacks.
9. When baking, use high-fiber flour such as whole wheat or oat flour.
10. Include legumes like beans, lentils, and chickpeas in your diet.
11. Read food labels carefully, and choose foods containing at least 6 grams of fiber per 100 grams.

As we continue to explore and learn, remember that listening to your body and making choices that align with your unique needs and preferences is essential. By incorporating these innovative ways to eat more fiber into your daily routine, you can nourish your body, support your gut health, and embark on a fulfilling and enjoyable dietary journey.

INCREASE YOUR FIBER INTAKE—BUT GRADUALLY

Embracing a fiber-rich diet can be a transformative step toward improving one's health and well-being. However, the transition may initially feel overwhelming for individuals accustomed to consuming processed foods.

While increasing your fiber intake is generally beneficial for your overall health, it is vital to be aware of potential side effects when making a sudden and significant increase in fiber consumption. These side effects are usually temporary and often resolve as your body adjusts to the change. Some potential side effects may include the following (Borkoles et al., 2022):

- **Digestive discomfort**: Rapidly increasing your fiber consumption can lead to bloating, gas, abdominal cramps, and an overall feeling of discomfort. This occurs because fiber absorbs water from the digestive tract, which can cause the stomach to expand and lead to temporary digestive issues.
- **Diarrhea or constipation**: A sudden influx of fiber can cause changes in your bowel movements. Some individuals may experience loose stools or diarrhea, whereas others may become constipated. Drinking plenty of water is essential when increasing your fiber intake to help maintain proper hydration and promote regular

bowel movements as your body gets used to your healthier diet.
- **Poor nutrient absorption**: High fiber intake can interfere with the absorption of certain minerals, such as zinc, iron, calcium, and magnesium. Although this is not typically a concern with a well-balanced diet, individuals with specific nutrient deficiencies or those relying heavily on fortified processed foods should monitor their nutrient intake.

It should be emphasized here that fiber absorbs water from the gut. Therefore, it is crucial to increase your fluid intake when you increase your fiber consumption. If there is insufficient water in your colon, your increased fiber intake may cause constipation, bloating, and abdominal discomfort instead of improving your bowel habits (Christian, 2022).

Note also that trying to reach the recommended daily intake of 30 grams of fiber immediately can lead to gut discomfort. Your digestive system needs time to adapt, and it may be overwhelmed by a sudden large influx of fiber. Therefore, it is much better to gradually increase your fiber intake over time to allow your body to adjust and minimize any potential for digestive discomfort.

In particular, your gut microbiota also needs its own time to adjust. Slowly increasing the amount of fiber you eat gives your gut microorganisms a chance to get used to the change. The beneficial microbes must grow in number to allow them to break down and use the extra fiber properly. In this way, your body can handle the increase in fiber without causing you any discomfort.

Everyone's needs are different, so it is a good idea to talk to a doctor or a nutrition expert, such as a registered dietitian, for advice tailored to you. They can help you determine the right amount of fiber to add to your diet and how to do it slowly and safely.

DOS AND DON'TS FOR INCREASING YOUR FIBER INTAKE

Do: Start With Small Amounts of Foods Containing Soluble Fiber

As a first step to increasing your fiber intake, you could begin your day with a bowl of oatmeal, eat lentil soup for lunch, add peas to your dinner, or snack on fruits such as apples and oranges during the day.

Do: Add Fiber-Rich Foods to Your Main Meals

Vegetables and whole grains are the easiest way to add fiber to your meals. As a general guideline, gradually work toward increasing the amount of vegetables on your plate until half of it is filled with vegetables at every meal.

Do: Start With the Fruits and Vegetables You Enjoy

If you are not a fan of fruit and vegetables and cannot bear the thought of eating more, start with the ones you actually enjoy. Include a manageable portion with every meal and start experimenting with different ones to increase the variety you eat slowly.

Do: Make Your Vegetables More Interesting

Find ways to make your vegetables more appealing. For example, you could add a little salt and a squeeze of lemon juice over your plain steamed broccoli, or you could sauté your spinach with sliced onion and garlic. Vegetables do not have to be plain and boring.

Do: Buy Frozen or Prepared Fruit and Vegetables

The easier it is to include fruit and vegetables in your meals, the more likely you are to eat them. The nutritional value of frozen fruit and vegetables compares favorably to that of fresh produce, and nothing is more straightforward than taking them out of the freezer and adding them to your meal. Using pre-prepared fresh vegetables also saves you time in the kitchen, making it easier to increase your intake of fiber-rich vegetables, however busy your schedule.

Don't: Make Sudden, Drastic Changes

Your digestive system needs time to adjust to a high fiber intake. As such, gradually increasing the amount of fiber you eat is better than rushing in. In other words, start small by swapping white bread for whole grain bread or making sure to include a portion of vegetables with your dinner. Then, every three to four days, you can add a little more until you are consuming the recommended 25 to 30 grams of fiber per day.

Don't: Rely Only on Fiber Supplements

Fiber supplements can be useful for increasing your fiber intake. However, it is best—and likely cheaper—to get your fiber from the food you eat. High-fiber foods are also usually rich in nutrients, promoting your overall health and well-being.

Don't: Eat Large Amounts of Legumes Straight Away

Legumes, such as beans and lentils, are high in fiber but can also cause gas and bloating if your body is not used to them. Begin by incorporating small portions and gradually increase this amount over time. It may also be helpful to start with split lentils that have had their hard outer husks removed to reduce the amount of fiber in your plant-based meals.

Don't: Include Too Many Gas-Forming Vegetables Too Soon

Cruciferous vegetables such as broccoli, cauliflower, and cabbage can cause excessive amounts of gas in the colon for some people. For that reason, introduce them into your diet in small portions over a period of time to minimize any discomfort they may cause.

Don't: Increase Your Fiber Intake Without Increasing Your Water Intake

Too much fiber and not enough water is a recipe for constipation and tummy aches. Therefore, as you start eating more fiber-rich foods, increasing the amount of water you drink is crucial. Start by including a glass of water before or after each meal.

Remember, everyone's tolerance to fiber varies, so just pay attention to your body's reactions and adjust your fiber intake accordingly. If you experience any symptoms associated with eating too much fiber, cut back, but do not give up. You cannot have a healthy gut without dietary fiber.

In this chapter, you have learned that fiber is crucial for your digestive tract and helps keep your gut healthy. Use the tips provided here to increase the amount of fiber in your diet slowly—but do not rush it. A sudden increase in fiber may be something of a shock to the system as it could overwhelm your gut microbiota. Give your microbial friends time to grow and adapt, letting them promote a healthy gut and improve your overall well-being.

In the next chapter, we will learn how having a balanced diet is essential for gut health. We will find out more about proteins, carbohydrates, healthy fats, vitamins, minerals, and all the different types of food that are good for your gut. I will show you how to put together a great mix of foods to support a healthy gut. So get ready to discover more about what to eat to keep your belly happy and healthy!

4

HACK #3: NOURISH YOUR GUT

A BALANCED DIET FOR OPTIMAL DIGESTION

> *"The doctor of the future will give no medicine, but will instruct his patient in the care of the human frame, in diet and in the cause and prevention of disease."*
>
> — THOMAS EDISON

Thomas Edison envisioned a future where doctors do not rely on drugs to treat the human body, instead focusing on nutrition to prevent and cure diseases. He emphasized the major role that nutrition plays in maintaining and improving our overall well-being (Nicklett & Kadell, 2013).

Your gut is crucial for digesting food, absorbing nutrients, and keeping your body healthy. But this is a two-way street—eating the right types of food is essential for helping your gut stay healthy and in good working condition.

Imagine your gut as a car engine. Just like a car needs the right fuel to run smoothly, your gut needs the right food to function properly. Conversely, an unhealthy diet can harm your gut in the same way as the wrong fuel can damage your car's engine. For example, consistently eating unhealthy and heavily processed foods can disrupt the natural balance in your digestive tract.

In this chapter, we will explore the critical role of a balanced diet in maintaining optimal gut health. Understanding the importance of nutrition will allow you to make informed decisions to support the health of your gut and entire body.

CHECK YOUR DIET

A poor diet can have severe consequences on your health. However, following a healthy diet can be challenging, especially in the United States and many other Western countries, where fast food and processed foods are everywhere. Almost half of all American adults suffer from chronic illnesses caused by their diet, with over 45% of deaths from heart disease, stroke, and diabetes being linked to what we eat.

What Is the Standard American Diet (SAD)?

The standard American diet, aptly abbreviated as SAD, consists primarily of processed foods containing large amounts of added sugars, unhealthy fats, and sodium, where the consumption of nutritious foods such as fruits, vegetables, whole grains, legumes, nuts, and seeds is neglected in favor of convenience and enhanced flavors. For people following this diet, typical meal options include pre-packaged foods containing artificial additives, flavors, and colors, fried foods, red meat, processed meats, sugary baked goods, refined grains, sugar-sweetened drinks, and dairy products.

Sadly (pun intended), the SAD is causing severe health problems for many Americans. Not only does it lead to weight gain, but it also increases the risk of chronic illnesses such as heart disease, stroke, diabetes, cancer, and fatty liver disease (Walker, 2015). Let us next look at some of the key problems with the SAD.

5 Major Problems With the SAD

1. **Sugar overload**: Sugar is hidden in many foods, even those marketed as healthy. Research shows that the more sugar you eat, the more you crave, and the average American consumes a shocking 77 grams (approximately 19 teaspoons) of it every single day. A high-sugar diet can lead to excessive blood sugar levels, insulin resistance, and an increased risk of developing diabetes (Witek et al., 2022).
2. **Processed foods**: Roughly 60% of the American diet consists of processed foods such as fast food, pre-packaged foods, frozen meals, sweets, cereals, canned soup, and sodas. These items offer little nutrition but are high in calories and contain large amounts of sodium, added sugars, and artificial flavors, colors, and preservatives.
3. **Lack of fruits and vegetables**: Fruits and vegetables are packed with vitamins, minerals, and dietary fiber, but many Americans simply do not eat enough. The recommended daily intake is 1.5–2 cups of fruits and 2–3 cups of vegetables, but very few people meet these goals (Lee et al., 2022).
4. **Lack of fiber**: Most Americans also do not consume enough dietary fiber, which, as you saw in the previous chapter, is crucial for gut health and regular bowel movements. The SAD includes large amounts of refined grain products like white rice and white flour, which are low in fiber and nutrients.

5. **Wrong fats**: Fast food and processed foods typically contain harmful trans fats that raise bad cholesterol and increase the risk of diabetes, heart disease, and stroke. However, your body needs good fats such as the omega-3 fatty acids found in salmon and walnuts, which are largely missing from the SAD.

Health Issues Caused by the SAD

The SAD is associated with numerous health concerns that potentially pose serious risks to overall well-being. Some of the main issues are presented below (Walker, 2015).

Obesity

The SAD is high in calories, unhealthy fats, and added sugars, all of which contribute to weight gain and obesity. Statistics suggest that 74% of adults in the United States are overweight or obese (Fryar et al., 2021). Obesity can increase the risk of a wide array of health conditions, including heart disease, type 2 diabetes, certain types of cancer, and joint problems.

The TV series *My 600-lb Life* documents the lives of individuals struggling with extreme obesity. The show often highlights the role of poor dietary choices and overconsumption of unhealthy foods in contributing to weight-related health issues.

Cardiovascular Disease

The SAD is high in saturated and trans fats, which can raise cholesterol levels and increase the risk of heart disease and stroke. Excessive sodium intake from processed foods can also contribute to high blood pressure, another known risk factor for cardiovascular issues (Grillo et al., 2019).

In the TV series *The Biggest Loser*, contestants often have underlying cardiovascular problems due to their unhealthy lifestyles. These individuals are encouraged to adopt healthier eating patterns to reduce their risk of heart disease.

Diabetes

The high content of refined carbohydrates and added sugars in the SAD can lead to insulin resistance and a greater risk of developing type 2 diabetes. This condition can have long-term negative consequences on both overall health and quality of life.

In the movie *Super Size Me*, filmmaker Morgan Spurlock performed a month-long experiment where he consumed only fast food to examine the harmful effects of a high-sugar, high-fat diet. Spurlock reported experiencing weight gain and mood swings and ultimately developed symptoms of prediabetes.

Nutrient Deficiencies

The SAD is lacking in essential nutrients such as vitamins, minerals, fiber, and antioxidants because of its limited inclusion of fruits, vegetables, and whole grains. This can lead to various nutrient deficiencies, poor immune function, and increased susceptibility to illnesses (CDC, 2022).

In the popular TV series *Breaking Bad*, one of the main characters, Jesse Pinkman, is depicted as having a poor diet that mainly consists of fast food and junk food. His overall health and well-being suffer as a result, reflecting the potential consequences of a nutrient-deficient diet.

Digestive Issues

The low fiber content of the SAD and its heavy reliance on processed foods can contribute to digestive problems such as constipation, IBS, and an imbalanced gut microbiota. These issues can impact overall digestion, nutrient absorption, and long-term gut health.

In the sitcom *Parks and Recreation*, the character Ron Swanson often showcases his love for a diet rich in meat and processed foods. While played for comedic effect, this portrayal neglects the potential digestive issues that can arise from a diet lacking in fiber and whole foods.

The Importance of a Balanced Diet for Gut Health

A balanced diet is critical for keeping your gut healthy and ensuring everything runs smoothly (Leeming et al., 2019). Here is why:

- A balanced diet includes fruits, vegetables, whole grains (such as brown rice and whole wheat bread), lean meats, and healthy fats. These foods contain essential nutrients, including vitamins, minerals, and dietary fiber, to help your digestive system function properly.
- As discussed in Chapter 3, fiber is a crucial part of food that your own body cannot break down. It helps move food and waste through your digestive system and keeps digestion running smoothly, thus feeding the good microbes in your gut and keeping you healthy.
- A balanced diet promotes the health of your gut microbiota. These essential microorganisms help break down the food you eat, make certain vitamins, and boost your immune system.
- A balanced diet can provide a good mix of digestive enzymes to support your body in breaking down food into smaller molecules so that the nutrients can be easily absorbed. Certain fruits, like pineapples and papayas,

themselves contain enzymes that may boost your digestive system.

A balanced diet means eating a mixture of healthy foods, consuming sufficient fiber, keeping your gut microbiota in balance, getting additional digestive enzymes from your food, drinking enough water, and avoiding unhealthy foods. Following a balanced diet will enable your gut to work well, promote nutrient absorption, and reduce the chances of tummy troubles.

CHOOSE WHOLE FOODS

What Is a Whole-Food Diet?

A whole-food diet is a way of eating that focuses on foods that are as close to their natural state as possible. It emphasizes the consumption of whole, unprocessed foods while minimizing the intake of processed foods (Song et al., 2022). Let us break down the key differences between whole foods and processed foods in simple terms.

Whole Foods

Whole foods are foods that have not been processed or refined, or those that have been processed to the minimum extent possible for consumption. Consequently, they retain all or most of their naturally occurring nutrients such as fiber and bioactive plant compounds (also known as phytochemicals), making them healthier options. Examples include fresh fruits and vegetables, whole grains like oats and brown rice, nuts, seeds, legumes such as beans and lentils, lean meats, and fish.

When you bring an apple or a carrot to work as a snack, you are eating a whole food in its natural form, just as it grows on a tree or in the ground.

Processed Foods

Processed foods, on the other hand, have been altered from their natural state through various processes, such as cooking, canning, freezing, or the addition of other ingredients. These foods often contain added sugars, unhealthy fats, and artificial additives. Processed foods include sugary cereals, packaged snacks, fast food, soda, processed meats like hot dogs and bacon, and pre-packaged meals (Albuquerque et al., 2022).

For instance, when you eat a bag of potato chips or a packaged dessert, you are consuming processed food. These have been modified from their natural state and contain added ingredients that are not as healthy for your body.

By choosing whole foods, you are giving your body the nutrients it needs in their natural form, without the added sugars, unhealthy fats, and artificial additives that can be detrimental to your health.

What Are the Potential Benefits of a Whole-Food Diet?

Whole foods are naturally rich in a diverse range of essential nutrients. Besides dietary fiber, vitamins, and minerals, whole foods often contain antioxidants, which help protect our bodies from cell damage caused by reactive molecules called free radicals, and phytochemicals, natural plant-derived compounds that possess potent antioxidant, anti-inflammatory, and other properties. Consuming a diet high in nutrient-dense whole foods has been associated with a reduced risk of chronic diseases, improved immune function, and better overall health.

A whole-food diet, particularly one emphasizing plant-based foods, can positively impact heart health. Studies have shown that such a diet is associated with lower blood pressure, improved cholesterol levels, and a reduced risk of heart disease and stroke (Taylor, 2023).

Furthermore, a whole-food diet can support healthy weight management. Whole foods tend to be more filling and satisfying, leading to reduced calorie intake. Several studies have linked adherence to such a diet with positive health outcomes, such as lower body weight, reduced risk of obesity, and better weight control (Greger, 2020).

Eating a diet focused around whole plant-based foods has also been associated with a decreased risk of various chronic diseases, which has been ascribed to the abundance of antioxidants and phytochemicals in these foods. Research has shown that people following a whole-food diet have a lower risk of developing type 2 diabetes, certain types of cancer, and neurodegenerative disorders such as Alzheimer's disease (Bansal et al., 2021).

Moreover, whole foods, particularly those high in fiber, promote a healthy digestive system by preventing constipation, supporting a diverse and balanced gut microbiota, and reducing the risk of digestive disorders (Han & Xiao, 2020).

In summary, following a whole-food diet as part of a healthy lifestyle can lead to multiple benefits in terms of overall well-being and disease prevention:

1. Chronic disease prevention
2. Chronic disease management
3. Weight loss
4. Improved gastrointestinal health
5. A more robust immune system

Recommended Whole Foods for Better Gut Health

When it comes to having a healthy gut, it is crucial to focus on consistently eating a broad variety of nutritious foods. Some good options are listed below.

Probiotic-Rich Foods

Fermented foods like the examples below are an excellent way to naturally introduce beneficial bacteria into the gut, thus supporting digestion and gut health (Leeuwendaal et al., 2022).

- **Apple cider vinegar**: A type of vinegar produced by fermenting apple juice with yeast and bacteria.
- **Kefir**: A fermented milk drink made using kefir grains, living symbiotic colonies of beneficial yeast and bacteria.
- **Kimchi**: A Korean dish prepared from salted and fermented vegetables.
- **Kombucha**: A fermented drink made from black tea using a mixture of bacteria and yeast.
- **Miso**: A fermented soybean paste prepared using a fungus.
- **Sauerkraut**: A German dish made from salted and fermented cabbage.
- **Soft cheeses**: The bacteria used to make soft cheeses such as blue cheese are good probiotics.
- **Tempeh**: A traditional Indonesian food made by fermenting soybeans with a specific fungus.
- **Yogurt**: A fermented milk product obtained by introducing bacteria such as *Lactobacillus bulgaricus* and *Streptococcus thermophilus* to milk.

Fiber-Rich Prebiotic Foods

Dietary fiber is a prebiotic—an essential fuel for your gut microbiota. Some foods that are rich in prebiotic fiber are listed below (Davani-Davari et al., 2019):

- Almonds
- Artichokes
- Asparagus

- Bananas
- Broccoli
- Cabbages
- Cauliflowers
- Chickpeas
- Fresh fruits (such as apples, bananas, blackberries, blueberries, and raspberries)
- Onions
- Quinoa
- Sweet potatoes
- Whole grains

Other Foods Beneficial for Gut Health

- **Avocados**: Avocados are rich in healthy fats, fiber, and vitamins and can promote gut health (Thompson et al., 2021).
- **Bone broth**: While not a cure-all, homemade bone broth can be easy to digest and provides beneficial nutrients (Mar-Solís et al., 2021).
- **Chicory root**: The root of this plant is rich in the prebiotic carbohydrate inulin and minerals that support gut health (Pouille et al., 2022).
- **Ginger and ginger beer**: Ginger has soothing effects on digestion, while ginger beer is a probiotic-filled soda that can be a better choice than other sweet carbonated beverages (Wang et al., 2021).
- **Sprouted grains**: These are grains or seeds that have been soaked in water and allowed to sprout, increasing their nutritional value and digestibility (Benincasa et al., 2019).

By incorporating these foods into your diet, you can take steps toward improving your gut health and digestion. Remember that a balanced diet with whole fruits and vegetables benefits your overall health.

Foods to Avoid for Gut Health

By contrast, many commonly eaten foods can cause an imbalance in your gut microbiota and promote inflammation in your digestive tract. As a result, eating a diet containing large amounts of these foods can damage your digestive health, negatively impacting your overall health and well-being. Some bad options of foods that are better avoided or consumed only occasionally and in small quantities are given below.

Acidic Foods

Highly acidic foods like citrus fruits, tomatoes, and vinegar can irritate the gut lining and worsen symptoms for individuals with conditions such as acid reflux or gastritis. However, these foods are generally well tolerated by most people and can provide health benefits (Newberry & Lynch, 2019).

Artificial Sweeteners

Some artificial sweeteners, such as aspartame and sucralose, can disrupt the gut microbiota and promote the growth of unhealthy bacteria. They may also contribute to gut inflammation and digestive issues (Ruiz-Ojeda et al., 2019).

Dairy Products

Dairy products can cause digestive issues such as bloating, gas, and diarrhea, especially for individuals who are lactose intolerant or otherwise sensitive to dairy. Some people may also experience an inflammatory response to the proteins found in dairy products (Aslam et al., 2020).

Fried Foods

Fried foods are often high in unhealthy fats and can lead to inflammation in the gut. They are also harder to digest and can contribute to digestive discomfort and irritation (Qi, 2021).

Gluten

For individuals with celiac disease or gluten sensitivity, consuming gluten-containing foods can cause the intestinal lining to become inflamed and damaged. However, most people can tolerate gluten without adverse effects (Garcia-Mazcorro et al., 2018).

Processed Foods

Processed foods typically contain additives, preservatives, and other artificial ingredients that can disrupt the gut microbiota and lead to inflammation. Moreover, they are often low in fiber and essential nutrients, thus negatively impacting gut health (Albuquerque et al., 2022).

Red Meat

Excessive intake of red meat has been associated with an increased risk of certain gut disorders, such as colorectal cancer. Red meat is also harder to digest than some other protein sources and can lead to inflammation in the gut (Wang et al., 2021).

Refined Grains

Refined grains lack much of the fiber and other nutrients found in whole grains because of the removal of the bran and germ during the milling process. Consequently, they can contribute to constipation and an imbalanced and less diverse gut microbiota (Jones et al., 2020).

Refined Sugars

Excessive consumption of refined sugars can disrupt the gut microbiota, promote the growth of harmful bacteria, and lead to inflammation in the gut. It can also contribute to conditions such as an overgrowth of *Candida*, a type of yeast found in the gut (Garcia et al., 2022).

Saturated Fats

A high intake of saturated fats, which are commonly found in fatty meats and full-fat dairy products, can lead to gut inflammation and disrupt the gut microbiota. It may also increase the risk of conditions such as inflammatory bowel disease (IBD) and metabolic syndrome (Zhang & Yang, 2016).

Soy

Some individuals may be sensitive or intolerant to soy products, which can cause digestive issues such as bloating, gas, and diarrhea. However, it is important to note that soy is well tolerated by most people and can be part of a healthy diet (Belobrajdic et al., 2023).

Spicy Foods

Spicy foods can sometimes irritate the digestive system, especially for individuals with conditions such as acid reflux, stomach ulcers, or IBS. They may also exacerbate symptoms such as heartburn, abdominal pain, and diarrhea (McDonald, 2018).

Tap Water

Depending on how water is treated in the area where you live, tap water may contain chlorine, fluoride, and other substances that can disrupt the gut microbiota. As such, consuming filtered or purified water is recommended whenever possible (Vanhaecke et al., 2022).

MINDFUL EATING

What Is Mindful Eating?

Mindful eating is a practice that involves devoting complete attention to the experience of eating, focusing on the sensations, thoughts, and emotions that arise during a meal. It encourages individuals to develop a deeper connection with their food, their body, and the act of eating (Nelson, 2017).

How Does It Work?

The goal of mindful eating is to maintain awareness of the present moment and cultivate a nonjudgmental attitude toward food and eating. Instead of rushing through your meals or eating on autopilot, mindful eating encourages you to slow down, savor each bite, and be fully present during the eating process.

Benefits of Mindful Eating

Mindful eating helps us choose more nutritious foods to improve our eating habits. It also allows us to enjoy and appreciate our food more, even while consuming smaller amounts. Eating mindfully can improve your digestion because you will eat more slowly and chew your food more thoroughly. In addition, it supports weight management techniques and allows you to make more unrestricted choices by refocusing on your eating habits. When you take the time to consider exactly what you are eating, you become more aware of where your food comes from, which in turn helps you appreciate everyone involved in its production. It is like "reformatting your brain's hard drive" (Cleveland Clinic, 2022).

Mindful eating helps you prevent overeating by tuning in to your body's hunger and fullness cues, thus promoting a healthier relationship with food. You become more attuned to your body's needs and preferences, leaving you better able to identify the types of foods that make you feel energized, nourished, and satisfied, which allows you to make your food choices accordingly.

This practice encourages individuals to engage all of their senses while eating. As a result, you can better appreciate the aromas, tastes, and textures of your food, leading to a more pleasurable eating experience. It also helps you become more aware of your emotions and triggers related to food, enabling you to make conscious choices rather than reacting impulsively.

8 Steps to Mindful Eating

With these benefits in mind, it helps to have some guidelines to get you started. Here are eight practical steps recommended by Harvard Health (2016a) to help you practice mindful eating:

1. **Begin with your shopping list**: Before heading to the grocery store, create a shopping list of nutritious foods you enjoy. This helps you to make conscious choices and avoid impulse purchases.
2. **Come to the table with an appetite—but not when ravenously hungry**: It is best to eat when you are moderately hungry rather than famished. This allows you to better appreciate your food and make mindful choices.
3. **Start with a small portion**: Serve yourself a small portion of food to start. You can always get more if you are still hungry after. This helps you avoid overeating and encourages you to be more mindful of portion sizes.
4. **Appreciate your food**: Take a moment to appreciate the colors, textures, and aromas of your meal. This can assist

with cultivating a sense of gratitude and enhance your enjoyment of your food.
5. **Bring all your senses to the meal**: Engage your senses fully while eating. Notice the taste, texture, and temperature of each bite, and pay attention to the sounds and smells of your food. This helps you stay present and fully experience the meal.
6. **Take small bites**: Instead of rushing through your meal, take small bites. Focus on thoroughly chewing and savoring each one. This allows you to taste your food better and enjoy its flavors.
7. **Chew thoroughly**: Chew your food thoroughly before swallowing. This aids in digestion and helps you recognize feelings of fullness more accurately. It also gives you time to appreciate the flavors and textures of your meal.
8. **Eat slowly**: Take the time to eat slowly and mindfully by putting your utensils down between bites and taking breaks to breathe and relax. This gives your body time to register feelings of satisfaction and prevents overeating.

Start incorporating these eight steps gradually into your meals. With practice, you will develop a deeper connection with your food and cultivate a healthier relationship with eating.

In this chapter, we have learned that maintaining a balanced diet is crucial for a healthy gut. A balanced diet supports digestion, nutrient absorption, and a robust immune system. In the next chapter, we will explore the gut–brain connection. We will discuss how stress and sleep affect your gut health and learn practical tips for managing stress and improving sleep to support a healthy gut. Taking care of your mind and body is essential for a happy gut.

MAKE A DIFFERENCE WITH YOUR REVIEW

UNLOCK THE POWER OF GENEROSITY

"Helping one person might not change the world, but it could change the world for one person."

— ANONYMOUS

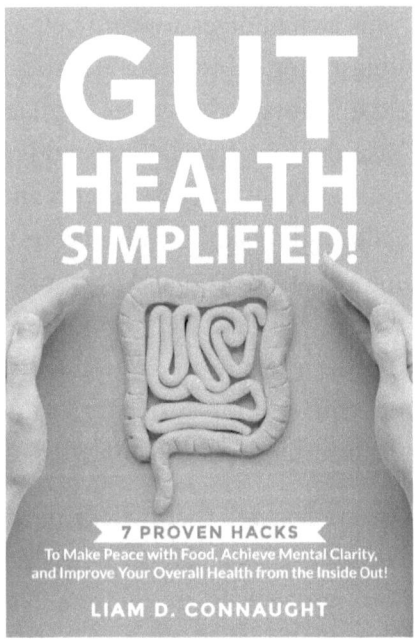

People who give without expecting anything in return often find more joy, live longer, and even feel more successful. So, during our time together, let's aim for that happiness.

I have a question for you:

Would you help someone you've never met, even if no one knew you did it?

Who is this person, you ask? They are like you once were: eager to learn, wanting to make a difference, and needing guidance on their journey.

My mission is to make **Gut Health** simple and accessible for everyone. Everything I do stems from that mission. And the only way for me to reach everyone is with your help.

This is where you come in. Most people do judge a book by its cover (and its reviews). So, on behalf of someone who is struggling with their gut health, here is my ask:

Please help that person by leaving this book a review.

Your gift costs no money and less than 60 seconds of your time, but it could change a fellow reader's life forever. Your review could help:

- One more person understand their gut health.
- One more family eat healthier meals.
- One more student excel in their studies.
- One more friend feel better every day.
- One more dream come true.

To feel great about helping someone and making a real difference, all you have to do is leave a review. It takes less than one minute. Please consider leaving a review on whichever platform you purchased it from! You'll show other readers where they can find the information they're seeking and help spread the word about gut health.

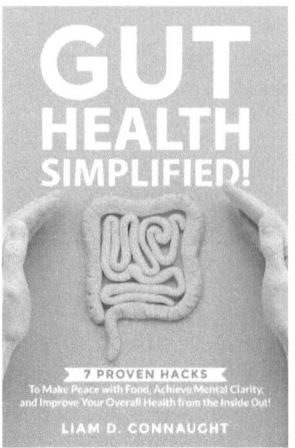

Thank you for your help. Gut health is kept alive when we share what we've learned—and you're helping me do just that.

If you enjoy helping others, you're my kind of person. Welcome to the club—you're one of us.

I'm excited to help you make peace with food, achieve mental clarity, and improve your overall health from the inside out. You'll love the strategies I'm about to share in the coming chapters.

Thank you from the bottom of my heart. Now, back to our regularly scheduled programming.

—Your biggest fan, Liam D. Connaught

P.S. Fun fact: Helping others not only feels good but also makes you feel more valuable. If you think this book will help someone you know, please share it with them.

5

HACK #4: CHILL OUT

REDUCE STRESS AND IMPROVE SLEEP FOR A HAPPIER GUT

 "Your gut is not Las Vegas. What happens in the gut does not stay in the gut."

— ALESSIO FASANO, MD, MASSACHUSETTS GENERAL HOSPITAL, USA

Stress affects everyone, irrespective of background or life situation. While its impact on our mental and emotional well-being may be directly evident, it can also profoundly influence the intricate ecosystem residing within our digestive system—the gut microbiota.

Similarly, unlike Las Vegas, what happens in your gut does not just stay there. It also affects your entire body, including your brain.

Remember the gut–brain connection we talked about in Chapter 1? It makes sense that if your digestive system is not well, it may have knock-on effects on your brain, influencing how you think and feel. In turn, stress can disrupt the balance of good and bad microbes in your digestive tract and even lead to a leaky gut. This leakiness can cause various problems in not only your digestive system but other parts of your body too.

Getting good sleep is not only good for your brain and overall health but also crucial for your digestive health. If you are not sleeping well, you may suffer from daytime tiredness, a low mood, and brain fog. A lack of sleep can also affect the gut microbiota balance, resulting in inflammation.

Remember that bustling community of tiny living microorganisms that make up your gut microbiota, a team of valuable workers helping to ensure your food is adequately digested and boosting your immune system? Stress can be compared to a tidal wave crashing through this community, disrupting its natural balance by killing off some beneficial microbes and allowing harmful ones to flourish. This shift upsets the harmony in your gut.

It is like changing the recipe of a dish you love. If you add too much of one ingredient and too little of another, the outcome will not taste the same. Similarly, when the microbial balance in your gut changes, it can throw off your entire digestive system. As you may have found out, this disruption can lead to digestive issues, bloating, or irregular bathroom visits. Its impact, however, reaches further than your gut.

Because your gut and brain are engaged in a constant two-way conversation, when your gut is upset owing to stress, it sends signals to your brain that affect your mood and thoughts.

Here is the good news: By finding ways to manage stress, such as deep breathing, meditation, or spending time doing activities you enjoy, you can help keep the balance of your gut microbiota in check. When the microbial community in your gut is happy and balanced, your digestive system tends to be happier and your brain will also function better!

HOW STRESS AFFECTS GUT HEALTH

Have you ever felt those "butterflies" in your stomach when you are nervous? Stress can impact your stomach as well as the rest of your digestive system. When you are under stress, your brain triggers your sympathetic nervous system, which activates your fight-or-flight mode. This system focuses on protecting you from immediate danger, part of which means slowing down digestion so that your body's resources can be better invested elsewhere. This delay can lead to stomach aches, indigestion, heartburn, and nausea (Leigh et al., 2023).

Interestingly, stress also revs up activity in the large intestine, potentially causing an urgent need to go to the bathroom. This can develop into a cycle—stress causes digestive symptoms, and those symptoms in turn create more stress. Chronic stress can also make existing gastrointestinal issues worse.

You can, however, help your gut by managing stress. To do this, you must activate your parasympathetic nervous system, your body's rest-and-digest response. This counteracts the effects of your sympathetic nervous system (Tindle & Tadi, n.d.).

The Gut–Brain Connection: A Biological Synchrony

Let us think about the two main characters involved in this gut–brain connection:

Your gut: As we know, this means your digestive system, including your stomach, your intestines, and the bustling community of microorganisms that help process the food you eat.

Your brain: This is the control center of your body, responsible for thinking, feeling, and making decisions.

Now let us get to the connection part:

Neurons: Your brain has numerous nerve cells called neurons—approximately 86 billion of them—which help transmit messages. Similarly, your gut "has a nervous system with more neurotransmitters than the brain's central nervous system," according to Tracey Torosian, PhD, of Henry Ford Health, such that it is often referred to as a "second brain" (Henry Ford Health, n.d.).

Have you ever heard someone say "I have a gut feeling about this"? Well, it is not just a saying—it is science! Here is how your gut communicates with your brain:

Gut bacteria: You have trillions of microorganisms living in your gut. In addition to helping digest food, these produce chemicals that can affect your mood and brain.

Hormones: Your gut releases hormones that can travel to your brain through your bloodstream and influence your emotions and thoughts.

When your gut talks, your brain listens, and vice versa! If your gut microbiota is happy, you are more likely to feel happy too. Conversely, a stressed brain can upset your gut. This is a two-way street—stress can interfere with your gut, and an unhappy gut can make you feel more stressed.

Sometimes, however, the gut–brain connection can get out of sync, contributing to problems such as depression or anxiety. If you are experiencing persistent issues, it is essential to talk to a healthcare professional for guidance. Your gut and brain are a dynamic duo, influencing each other in ways you might not have imagined. By taking care of both your gut and your brain, you can enhance your overall health and well-being (Foster et al., 2017).

Real-Life Consequences: Stress and Gastrointestinal Disorders

Stress exerts significant consequences on the gut and may trigger or exacerbate various gastrointestinal disorders. This highlights the profound impact that psychological factors can have on physical health. Some examples of common gastrointestinal disorders affected by stress are given below.

Irritable Bowel Syndrome (IBS)

Exacerbation of symptoms: Stress is a well-known trigger for the symptoms of IBS, such as abdominal pain, bloating, diarrhea, and constipation (Chang, 2011).

Real-life example: A person with IBS may experience flare-ups of their symptoms during periods of high stress, like work deadlines or a personal crisis.

Inflammatory Bowel Disease (IBD)

Exacerbation of symptoms: Chronic stress can increase inflammation and disease activity in individuals with Crohn's disease or ulcerative colitis, the two main forms of IBD (Ge et al., 2022).

Real-life example: A person with Crohn's disease may experience more frequent and severe flare-ups during stressful life events.

Gastroesophageal Reflux Disease (GERD)

Exacerbation of symptoms: Stress can increase stomach acid production and relax the lower esophageal sphincter between the esophagus and stomach, leading to more frequent heartburn and acid reflux (Song et al., 2012).

Real-life example: Someone with GERD may find that stress from a demanding job increases the severity and frequency of their episodes of heartburn.

Functional Dyspepsia

Exacerbation of symptoms: Stress can aggravate the symptoms of functional dyspepsia—a recurring upset stomach with no obvious cause. These symptoms include feeling full too soon, bloating, and discomfort in the upper abdomen (Nam et al., 2018).

Real-life example: A person with functional dyspepsia may notice that their symptoms worsen when they are under stress, especially during social gatherings or work-related events.

Peptic Ulcer Disease

Exacerbation of symptoms: Although stress alone does not directly cause ulcers, it can increase the risk of their development by impacting the stomach's protective mechanisms and making the stomach lining more susceptible to acid-mediated damage (Lee et al., 2017).

Real-life example: An individual exposed to chronic stress may be more vulnerable to developing peptic ulcers, especially if they have other risk factors such as *Helicobacter pylori* infection or the use of non-steroidal anti-inflammatory drugs.

Gastrointestinal Motility Disorders

Exacerbation of symptoms: Stress can slow down the movement of food through the digestive tract, leading to symptoms like nausea, vomiting, and abdominal pain (Stengel & Taché, 2009).

Real-life example: A person with gastroparesis, a condition involving delayed emptying of the stomach due to a change in the contraction of the stomach muscles, may notice that their symptoms worsen during stressful periods, making it even more challenging to manage their condition.

Changes in Gut Microbiota

Exacerbation of symptoms: Chronic stress can disrupt the balance between beneficial and harmful gut microbes, potentially contributing to gastrointestinal disorders or aggravating existing conditions (Gao et al., 2022).

Real-life example: Research has shown that individuals under chronic stress may experience alterations in their gut microbiota, which can impact digestion and overall health.

It is crucial to understand that the gut–brain connection is bidirectional. While stress can worsen gastrointestinal symptoms, digestive problems can also lead to increased stress and anxiety, creating a vicious cycle.

BENEFITS OF STRESS MANAGEMENT TECHNIQUES FOR GUT HEALTH

The relationship between stress and the gut is well documented, and by reducing stress, people can positively impact their digestive system in several ways. Some of the key benefits of stress management techniques on gut health are outlined below (Gastrointestinal Society, n.d.-b).

Reduced Gastrointestinal Symptoms

Relaxation exercises and deep breathing can help calm your body's stress response. This can improve digestion and reduce symptoms of gastrointestinal disorders such as IBS, indigestion, and GERD.

Healthier Gut Microbiota

Chronic stress can disrupt the balance of beneficial and harmful microorganisms in your gut. Stress management techniques, including mindfulness and relaxation, can promote a healthier gut microbiota, which is associated with better overall gut health and reduced inflammation.

Better Nutrient Absorption

When your gut is less aggravated by stress, it functions more efficiently, allowing for improved absorption of essential vitamins, minerals, and other nutrients from your food.

Reduced Inflammation

Stress can trigger inflammation in your gut, leading to conditions such as IBD. Stress management techniques can help reduce chronic inflammation, leading to less damage to the digestive tract and improved gut health.

Improved Gastrointestinal Motility

Regular physical activity can promote healthy gastrointestinal motility. This means that food moves through your digestive tract at a normal rate, reducing the risk of conditions like constipation and gastroparesis.

Lower Risk of Stress-Induced Gut Disorders

By reducing stress, you may be less likely to develop conditions such as stomach ulcers and stress-induced gastritis (stomach inflammation).

Enhanced Immune Function

Stress management techniques may boost your immune function, and a strong immune system helps protect your gut from infections and maintain overall gut health.

Better Gut-Brain Communication

When stress is well managed, communication between your gut and brain improves. This can lead to a more balanced mood and help reduce depression and anxiety, which are closely linked to gut health. Remember that mood-regulating neurotransmitters such as serotonin and dopamine are produced in your gut and have a significant impact on your mental health.

Enhanced Quality of Life

Stress can reduce your quality of life by affecting your mood and making your digestive tract less reliable. It can also cause you to withdraw from social activities, make poor dietary choices, and follow a less active lifestyle. By contrast, when you feel good and your digestive system is working as it should, you are more likely to enjoy spending time with friends and family, and making healthy diet and lifestyle choices becomes much easier.

TIPS FOR MANAGING STRESS

Stress is the reaction of your mind and body to demanding circumstances. In our modern society, the hectic pace of work and personal life, the constant presence of technology, and the desire to maintain meaningful connections can sometimes make the stress feel almost overwhelming. Therefore, learning how to manage and reduce stress is crucial for improving your quality of life.

Selecting the best stress management technique for you is just as important as eating a healthy diet. Some people may enjoy taking time out with a cup of herbal tea and a good book, while others might prefer the natural high of an intense workout. Whatever you choose to do, it must help you relax—it is better to avoid activities you hate and that cause you even more stress.

Four useful ways to manage stress are focused exercise, meditation, deep breathing, and ensuring you get enough good-quality sleep. For the remainder of this chapter, we will dive into each of these.

Focused Exercise: Pilates

What Is Pilates?

Pilates is a fantastic way to reduce stress for several reasons (Lim & Park, 2019). It emphasizes mindful movements and precise control of the body, creating a meditative and calming experience. Concentrating on each movement and breath lets you stay in the present moment, allowing stressful thoughts to fade into the background.

Pilates also incorporates deep and rhythmic breathing, which activates your body's relaxation response. This controlled breathing promotes better oxygenation, reduces tension, and ultimately alleviates stress.

A significant additional benefit of Pilates is that the controlled movements enhance blood flow throughout your body, aiding in removing toxins and promoting overall relaxation.

Furthermore, Pilates exercises focus on stretching and elongating muscles. In doing so, they help release physical tension and can have a corresponding calming effect on the mind, thus reducing your stress levels.

Regularly practicing Pilates cultivates a heightened awareness of your body, enabling you to recognize and release areas of tension.

This self-awareness reduces stress as you become more in tune with your body's needs.

Gut-Friendly Pilates Exercises

Pilates exercises can be gentle on the digestive system, promoting gut health. However, proper form and alignment are essential to avoid injury and get the most benefit. If you are new to Pilates, consider taking classes with a certified instructor to ensure you are performing the exercises correctly.

Some Pilates exercises that are particularly friendly to your gut are given below.

Pelvic clocks: These exercises gently engage and mobilize your lower abdominal muscles, promoting digestion and reducing discomfort (Complete Pilates, n.d.-c):

1. Begin by lying on your back with your knees bent and feet flat on the floor.
2. Inhale as you tilt your pelvis toward your belly button (12 o'clock). Then, using your abdominal muscles, rotate your hips clockwise to the 3 o'clock position (left hip down).
3. Next, rotate your hips to the 6 o'clock position (pelvic bone tilted toward the floor).
4. Finally, rotate your hips to the 9 o'clock position (right hip down).
5. Return to the 12 o'clock position.
6. Repeat 8–10 times.

Bridge: Bridge exercises strengthen your core and promote overall body alignment, which can alleviate digestive discomfort (Sievers, 2021):

1. Lie on your back with your knees bent and feet flat on the floor, hip-width apart.
2. Inhale, engage your core by pulling your belly button toward your spine and lift your hips off the ground.
3. Exhale as you lower your hips back down to the starting position.
4. Repeat 8–10 times.

Roll-up: Roll-up exercises engage your abdominal muscles and promote intestinal motility, aiding digestion (Watts, n.d.):

1. Lie flat on the floor with your legs extended straight out in front of you and your arms extended to the ceiling.
2. Inhale as you lengthen your spine and engage your core.
3. Exhale and start raising the upper part of your body, bending at the hips and moving your chest toward your thighs, reaching for your toes with your fingertips.
4. Inhale again as you slowly roll back down, one vertebra at a time, and return to the starting position, using your abdominal muscles to control the movement.
5. Repeat 8–10 times.

Spine stretch forward: This exercise stretches the spine and promotes relaxation, potentially reducing stress-related digestive issues (Peak Pilates, 2019):

1. Sit with your legs extended straight in front of you with your toes pointing toward the ceiling.
2. Inhale as you lengthen your spine and reach forward with your arms.
3. Exhale as you fold forward at your hips, lowering your chest toward your thighs.

4. Pause, inhale, and slowly raise your body, one vertebra at a time.
5. Repeat 8–10 times, focusing on stretching and lengthening the spine.

Swan dive: Swan dive movements can help improve posture, reducing the risk of indigestion by minimizing pressure on the stomach (Complete Pilates, n.d.-b):

1. Lie facedown on your mat with your arms extended overhead.
2. Inhale, engage your abdominal muscles by pulling your belly button toward your spine and lift your head, chest, and arms off the mat.
3. Exhale as you slowly lower yourself back down to the starting position.
4. Repeat 8–10 times, emphasizing the extension of your spine.

Criss-cross (oblique twist): The criss-cross movement twists your abdomen, thus massaging your digestive tract (Complete Pilates, n.d.-a):

1. Lie on your back with your knees bent and hands behind your head.
2. Engage your abdominal muscles and lift your feet, head, neck, and shoulders off the mat.
3. Inhale and rotate your upper body to the right, bringing your left elbow toward your right knee.
4. Exhale and return to the center.
5. Do the same on the other side, bringing your right elbow toward your left knee.

6. Repeat the entire process 8–10 times, continuing to alternate sides in a controlled, twisting motion.

The saw: This is a bending, twisting movement that gently massages your gut (Physitrack, n.d.-a):

1. Sit with your legs extended in front of you, feet wide apart and arms stretched to the sides.
2. Inhale as you twist to the right, bending at the hips and reaching your left hand toward your right foot.
3. Exhale as you come back to the center.
4. Inhale and twist to the left, bending at the hips and reaching your right hand toward your left foot.
5. Exhale and return to the center.
6. Repeat 8–10 times on each side.

The hundred: This is a classic pilates exercise focusing on core strength (Physitrack, n.d.-b):

1. Lie on your back with your knees bent, feet flat on the floor, and arms at your sides.
2. Lift your head, neck, and shoulders off the mat.
3. Extend your legs straight and hover them above the ground.
4. Lift your arms and pump them up and down while breathing in for five counts and out for five counts.
5. Continue for 100 arm pumps while keeping your core engaged and your lower back on the mat.

Meditation

What Is Meditation?

Meditation entails focusing your mind on a particular object, thought, or activity to train your attention and awareness, promote relaxation, and achieve a mentally clear and emotionally calm state. Meditation has been practiced for thousands of years by various cultures and comes in numerous forms, but all share the common goal of quieting the mind and achieving a state of inner calm (National Center for Complementary and Integrative Health, 2022).

What Does Meditation Do?

Meditation offers a range of mental, emotional, and physical benefits. It helps moderate your body's stress response by decreasing the levels of stress hormones such as cortisol, thus promoting relaxation and a sense of calm.

Regular meditation can also enhance attention and concentration, making it easier to stay present and focused on tasks in daily life. In addition, it cultivates emotional awareness and resilience, which may help you manage negative emotions, anxiety, and depression.

A further benefit of meditation is enhanced self-awareness. It enables you to gain insights into your unique thought patterns, behaviors, and reactions, thereby promoting your personal growth.

Meditation can also improve your sleep quality by calming your mind, helping you fall asleep more quickly, and staying asleep throughout the night.

Furthermore, meditation has been used as a complementary

approach to manage chronic pain. It can bring relief by altering your perception of pain.

How Meditation Helps Reduce Stress

Meditation is a potent tool for stress reduction. Some of the key reasons for this are as follows (American Psychological Association, 2019):

- **Activation of the parasympathetic nervous system**: Meditation triggers your body's rest-and-digest state, countering the effects of the stress response. This reduces your heart rate, lowers your blood pressure, and decreases the production of stress hormones.
- **Calming of the mind**: Meditation encourages a mental shift away from stress-inducing thoughts and concerns, promoting mental clarity and emotional balance.
- **Enhanced resilience**: Regular meditation builds emotional resilience, enabling you to better cope with life's stressors.
- **Reduced muscle tension**: Meditation helps relax your muscles and release the physical tension that can accumulate during times of stress.

How to Meditate: Step-by-Step Instructions

Meditation can be practiced in various ways. The step-by-step guide given below explains how to meditate by focusing on your breathing (Carter & Carter, 2016). However, if you are new to meditation, you may find it easier to begin with guided meditation. This can be in the form of recordings or meditation apps, which provide a structured meditation session where a narrator guides you through the process and offers prompts for relaxation and focus.

Use the 10 steps below to begin your meditation practice.

1. **Find a comfortable space**: Choose a quiet and peaceful place where you will not be interrupted. This could be a corner of your room, a quiet bench at the park, or any serene location that suits you.
2. **Sit comfortably**: You can meditate in a chair with your feet flat on the ground or sit on a cushion or mat with your legs crossed. Ensure that your spine is straight but not tense.
3. **Relax your body**: Close your eyes and begin by taking a few deep breaths to release any physical tension. Allow your body to settle into a state of relaxation.
4. **Focus on your breath**: Observe the natural rhythm of your breathing without trying to control it. Pay attention to the sensation of each breath—how the air feels as it enters and leaves your nostrils and how your chest and abdomen rise and fall.
5. **Be mindful of your thoughts**: As you meditate, your mind may wander and thoughts may arise. This is perfectly normal. Instead of getting frustrated, acknowledge the thoughts without judgment and gently bring your focus back to your breath.
6. **Deepen your awareness**: Expand your awareness beyond your breath as you continue to inhale and exhale. Notice any sounds around you, the feeling of the ground beneath you, or the temperature of the air. Be fully present in the moment.
7. **Set a timer**: Decide on the duration of your meditation session. Begin with 5–10 minutes and gradually increase this time as you become more comfortable with the process. You may wish to use a timer or meditation app to keep track.

8. **Cultivate a nonjudgmental attitude**: Be patient with yourself during meditation. It is natural for the mind to wander. Your goal is not to eliminate thoughts but to gently bring your focus back to your chosen point of concentration.
9. **End mindfully**: When your meditation time is up, do not rush back into daily activities. Take a few deep breaths, slowly open your eyes, and transition back to your surroundings. Reflect on how you feel after the session.
10. **Be consistent**: Consistency is key for reaping the full benefits of meditation. Try to establish a regular meditation routine, ideally at the same time each day. Over time, this practice will become a valuable part of your daily life.

Meditation is a skill that develops with practice. It is completely normal to have days when meditation feels easier and others when it is more challenging. The key is to maintain a gentle and patient approach, and over time you will notice increased mental clarity, reduced stress, and improved overall well-being. Feel free to explore different meditation techniques and approaches to discover what resonates best with you, whether it is mindfulness meditation or another style that suits your needs and preferences.

Deep Breathing

What Is Deep Breathing?

Deep breathing, also known as diaphragmatic or abdominal breathing, involves taking slow, deliberate breaths by engaging the diaphragm muscle, which separates the chest and abdominal cavities. In contrast to shallow breathing, which involves quick, shallow breaths primarily using the chest, deep breathing focuses on slow, deep inhalations and exhalations, allowing for better oxygen exchange in the body (Harvard Health, 2016b).

Downsides of Shallow Breathing

Shallow breathing, which is typical during stressful situations or when individuals are not mindful of their breath, can have several adverse effects. In particular, it can trigger the body's stress response, leading to elevated levels of stress hormones such as cortisol alongside an increased heart rate.

Shallow breaths do not allow for optimal oxygen intake, potentially leading to fatigue and decreased cognitive function. In addition, they can contribute to muscle tension, especially in the neck and shoulders, resulting in discomfort and pain.

Finally, shallow breathing may disrupt normal digestive processes and contribute to gastrointestinal discomfort, including indigestion and IBS (Russo et al., 2017).

Potential Benefits of Deep Breathing

Deep breathing offers a range of physical, mental, and emotional benefits (Tavoian & Craighead, 2023):

1. It alleviates stress and reduces tension in the gut, thus stimulating better digestion.
2. It can help lower blood pressure and promote relaxation.
3. It helps calm the mind and reduce emotional reactions, thus improving overall psychological well-being.
4. It can improve cognitive function, making it easier to stay present and attentive.
5. If practiced before bedtime, it can enhance sleep quality by relaxing the body and mind.

How to Start Practicing Deep Breathing

Here are some step-by-step instructions for a basic deep breathing exercise (Harvard Health, 2016b):

1. **Find a comfortable position**: Sit or lie down in a comfortable position, with your back straight but not rigid and your shoulders relaxed.
2. **Place your hands**: Rest your hands on your abdomen, just below your ribcage, so you can feel the rise and fall of your tummy as you breathe.
3. **Inhale slowly**: Take in a slow, deep breath through your nose. Feel your abdomen rise as you fill your lungs with air. Aim to inhale for approximately 4–6 seconds.
4. **Exhale slowly**: Exhale slowly and completely through your mouth. As you exhale, feel your abdomen fall. Again, aim to exhale for about 4–6 seconds.
5. **Repeat**: Continue this deep breathing pattern for several breaths, focusing each time on the rise and fall of your abdomen.
6. **Maintain a rhythm**: Establish a rhythm that feels comfortable for you. As you become more comfortable with the technique, gradually increase the duration of your inhalations and exhalations.
7. **Stay present**: If your mind starts to wander, gently bring your focus back to your breath and the sensation of rising and falling in your abdomen.
8. **Practice regularly**: Incorporate deep breathing into your daily routine, especially during stressful or anxious moments.

By regularly practicing deep breathing, you can experience its numerous benefits and promote your overall well-being.

High-Quality Sleep

A lack of good sleep can significantly impact your gut health, leading to various digestive and overall health issues (Chattu et al., 2019). Sleep deprivation often triggers increased stress levels because your body needs rest to recover and repair. This elevated stress may then disrupt the gut microbiota, potentially resulting in gastrointestinal problems.

In addition, making healthy food choices becomes more challenging when you are deprived of sleep. You may end up opting for sugary, high-fat, or processed foods instead of healthy home-cooked meals, thus unbalancing your gut microbiota and contributing to inflammation in your digestive tract.

Sleep is also crucial for regulating the hormones that influence your appetite and metabolism. For example, sleep deprivation can cause imbalances in hormones like leptin and ghrelin, which control hunger and fullness, potentially leading to overeating and unhealthy weight gain.

Furthermore, sleep deprivation may contribute to increased intestinal permeability and the development of a leaky gut. This condition allows harmful substances to pass through the intestinal lining and enter the bloodstream, triggering widespread inflammation as well as digestive discomfort.

Moreover, a lack of sleep can relax the lower esophageal sphincter, allowing stomach acid to flow back into the esophagus, leading to acid reflux, heartburn, and indigestion.

Staying up too late and eating too close to bedtime can also disrupt the body's natural digestion and restorative processes during sleep. This can result in discomfort, acid reflux, and disturbed sleep patterns, which can negatively affect gut health.

Benefits of High-Quality Sleep for Gut Health

Getting good sleep is essential for maintaining optimal gut health and overall well-being. Here are some benefits of high-quality sleep (Wu et al., 2023):

- **Maintains a healthy gut microbiota**: Getting enough sleep helps promote good diversity and stability in your gut microbiota.
- **Reduces inflammation**: Ensuring an adequate amount of high-quality sleep helps reduce inflammation in your body, including the gut, which is crucial for digestive comfort.
- **Boosts digestion**: A well-rested body can digest food more efficiently, which enables better nutrient absorption and overall digestive health.
- **Regulates hormones**: Quality sleep helps regulate hormones related to your appetite, metabolism, and stress, supporting your overall well-being.
- **Enhances gut–brain communication**: Restorative sleep enhances the communication between your gut and brain, contributing to mental clarity and emotional well-being.

Consequently, prioritizing high-quality sleep is essential for maintaining good gut health. It helps reduce stress, supports healthy dietary choices, regulates hormones, and prevents digestive disturbances. By recognizing the importance of sleep in your digestive health, you can take proactive steps to improve your overall well-being and enhance the health of your gut microbiota.

Tips for Improving Sleep Quality

While some of the suggestions below may seem obvious, taking the necessary steps to get a good night's sleep is often not a priority owing to the busyness of everyday life. As a result, feeling tired and stressed has unfortunately become the norm for many people.

Use the tips below to establish good sleep hygiene and a bedtime routine that helps you fall asleep and stay asleep so that you feel rested the next day (Chow, 2022).

1. **Increase bright light exposure in the morning**: Exposure to natural light during the day helps regulate your body's internal clock and enhances alertness. Spend time outdoors, especially in the morning, to promote better sleep at night.
2. **Reduce blue light exposure in the evening**: Blue light from screens like those of your smartphone, computer, and TV can interfere with your sleep/wake cycle. Minimize your screen time in the evening or use blue-light-blocking glasses, and try to switch off your devices at least one hour before bedtime.
3. **Avoid caffeine late in the day**: Caffeine is a stimulant that can disrupt sleep. Avoid tea, coffee, colas, and foods such as chocolate in the afternoon and evening.
4. **Avoid daytime naps**: While short, occasional naps can be refreshing, long or irregular napping during the day can interfere with nighttime sleep. If daytime naps are necessary, it is better to limit them to 20–30 minutes.
5. **Establish a consistent sleep/wake cycle**: Maintain a regular sleep schedule, even on weekends. In other words, go to bed and wake up at the same time every day. This may be difficult at first, but consistency helps regulate your body's internal clock, making it easier to fall asleep and wake up as you become accustomed to your new routine.

6. **Avoid alcohol**: Although alcohol can make it easier to fall asleep, it can also disrupt sleep patterns and reduce the overall quality of your sleep. Limit your alcohol intake, especially in the hours leading up to bedtime.
7. **Optimize your bedroom environment**: Create a relaxing environment in your bedroom by keeping it dark and quiet. Consider using blackout curtains and white noise machines if needed.
8. **Keep your bedroom cool**: A cooler bedroom temperature (around 65–70°F or 18–21°C) is generally more conducive to sleep. Adjust your thermostat accordingly. If you do not have air conditioning, use a fan to keep your bedroom cool.
9. **Eat your last meal 2–3 hours before bedtime**: Consuming large or spicy meals close to bedtime can lead to discomfort and indigestion. Finish eating at least 2–3 hours before sleep.
10. **Relax and clear your mind in the evening**: Engage in relaxing activities before bedtime, such as reading, gentle stretching, or deep breathing exercises. These help calm the mind and prepare you for sleep.
11. **Take a warm bath or shower**: A warm bath or shower in the evening can help you relax and signal to your body that it is time to wind down for sleep. It also leads to a slight decrease in your body temperature, which promotes good sleep.
12. **Rule out a sleep disorder**: If you consistently have trouble sleeping despite practicing good sleep hygiene, consult a healthcare professional to rule out underlying sleep disorders such as sleep apnea and insomnia.
13. **Get a comfortable bed, mattress, and pillow**: Your sleep environment should be comfortable. Invest in a quality mattress and pillow that support your sleeping posture.

14. **Exercise regularly**: Regular physical activity can improve your sleep quality. However, avoid vigorous exercise close to bedtime, as it may energize you and make it harder to fall asleep.
15. **Do not drink too much liquid before bed**: Limit your fluid intake in the evening to prevent nighttime awakenings for bathroom trips. Drink fluids earlier in the day to stay well hydrated.

By incorporating these tips into your daily routine, you can enhance your sleep quality and overall well-being. Remember that everyone's sleep needs are unique, so it may take some experimentation to determine the best strategies for you.

In this chapter, we have learned that stress and sleep quality can significantly impact our gut health by disrupting the balance of the gut microbiota. We have discussed ways to deal with stress and discovered how to sleep better, like relaxing and creating a cozy sleep environment.

In the next chapter, we will explore how regular physical activity can make your gut microbiota and brain even happier. You will find out how simple activities in your daily life can improve your digestion and overall well-being with some easy tips on staying active and keeping your gut feeling great. So, get ready to boost your gut health by adding some movement to your routine!

HACK #5: MOVE IT

HOW EXERCISE CAN IMPROVE YOUR GUT HEALTH

 "Physical fitness is not only one of the most important keys to a healthy body, it is the basis of dynamic and creative intellectual activity."

— JOHN F. KENNEDY

In today's world, many of us spend most of our day at a desk, sitting for 6–8 hours at a time. In addition, instead of walking or cycling to work, we hop in the car, catch a bus, or use the train. Therefore, exploring ways to incorporate movement into our daily routines has become more crucial than ever.

A lack of physical activity can adversely affect your digestive system and general well-being. Spending long hours sitting can slow down the natural movement of your intestines, potentially leading to issues including constipation and discomfort. Furthermore, reduced physical activity may negatively impact the diversity and health of your gut microbiota.

Making the effort to incorporate movement into your daily life can help avoid these problems. Regular exercise, even in moderate amounts, can enhance your gut health. Simple practices like taking short breaks to stand up, stretch, or go for a quick walk can stimulate blood flow throughout your body and support the natural contractions of the intestines. These movements can aid in the smoother passage of food through the digestive tract, reducing the likelihood of digestive discomfort.

Physical activity promotes a diverse and balanced gut microbiota and is essential for efficient digestion and nutrient absorption. It can also help regulate inflammation in the gut, contributing to a healthier digestive system overall.

In this chapter, I aim to help you understand how moving around can improve your gut health. I will also include easy tips on how to sneak exercise into your everyday life.

HOW MOVEMENT AFFECTS GUT HEALTH

How Sitting Too Long Influences Your Gut

When you spend a lot of time sitting, especially in front of a computer or TV, your digestion slows down. The lack of movement causes your blood to move more sluggishly through the blood vessels in your body. This includes the blood vessels that carry oxygenated blood to your digestive system and nutrients from your gut to the cells throughout your body that need energy, vitamins, and minerals to function. When your blood flow slows down, it makes your digestive system sluggish too. Muscle contractions are also affected, delaying the movement of food through the intestines.

Furthermore, sitting too much can impact the community of microorganisms living in your gut. It may disrupt the balance of these microbes, which, alongside other digestive problems, can lead to a weaker immune system.

Habitually sitting for long periods can also cause weight gain and obesity, harming your gut health. As such, finding ways to move more during the day is essential to keep your gut happy and healthy.

How Physical Activity Promotes Digestion and a Healthy Gut Microbiota

Physical activity plays a major role in promoting digestion and maintaining a healthy gut microbiota. Recent research indicates that exercise can have an array of positive effects on your gut health, including the following six examples (Monda et al., 2017):

1. Exercise stimulates the muscles in your digestive tract, promoting more regular and efficient bowel movements. This can help prevent issues like constipation and abdominal discomfort.
2. Regular activity can enhance the diversity and balance of your gut microbiota. It encourages the growth of beneficial microbial species, creating a healthier gut environment.
3. Exercise can boost your immune system as the development of beneficial microbes in your gut plays a crucial role in immune function. This, in turn, helps your body better defend itself against infections and diseases.
4. Physical activity can increase your metabolic rate, helping your body use energy from food more efficiently and promoting better nutrient absorption.

5. As we saw in Chapter 5, exercise is a well-known stress reducer. High-stress levels can disrupt the balance of your gut microbiota and lead to digestive discomfort, so lowering stress levels will inevitably have a positive impact on your gut health.
6. Regular exercise is associated with a reduced risk of colon cancer. By promoting regular bowel movements, exercise decreases inflammation in the colon, potentially modifying the composition of the gut microbiota in a way that is less conducive to cancer development.

EXERCISES TO SUPPORT YOUR GUT HEALTH

Specific exercises can help your gut stay in tip-top shape. Let us explore some easy exercises that support gut health (Boytar et al., 2023).

Jogging

Jogging gets your body moving and your heart pumping. It also helps your digestive system work better by stimulating muscle contractions in the intestines, thus promoting the movement of food and waste through your digestive tract. In other words, the simple act of jogging slowly around a park and enjoying the fresh air can actively improve your gut!

Walking

Walking is one of the most accessible forms of exercise, requiring no special equipment. A brisk walk is great for your overall health, including your digestion. Even a leisurely stroll through your neighborhood will help your gut stay in good shape.

Swimming

Swimming is a fun and refreshing way to exercise your whole body and can help digestion. Your abdominal muscles work hard while swimming, gently massaging your gut and promoting digestion and food movement through your intestines.

Cycling

When you pedal a bike, either in a gym or outside, the workout for both your legs and abdominal muscles can help keep your digestive system happy.

Elliptical Trainer

An elliptical machine (a fancy exercise device found at the gym) is gentle on your joints and can give you a good workout. You move your legs in a smooth, circular motion, and your abdominal muscles work at the same time to keep you upright, helping your gut stay healthy.

Pilates

As we learned in Chapter 5, Pilates is a workout that focuses on your core muscles, including those around your digestive tract. Strengthening these muscles can support your digestion. When you practice Pilates exercises on a mat or with special equipment, you work on your core strength, which can benefit your gut health.

So, whether you are jogging through the park, swimming in the pool, or simply walking, these exercises can help keep your gut in good working order. Not only are you using the large muscles of your arms, legs, and back, which boosts your metabolism, but your abdominal muscles are getting a workout too, making sure your digestive system is operating efficiently.

TIPS FOR MAKING YOUR EXERCISE ROUTINE MORE GUT-FRIENDLY

Exercise can be the key to keeping your gut in top form. In this part of the book, I will walk you through some useful tips to help you optimize your exercise routine for maximum gut health. From focusing on cardiovascular workouts to maintaining consistency, starting small, embracing the outdoors, and paying attention to your nutrition, let us get moving toward a healthier gut.

1. **Focus on cardio**: Cardiovascular exercises are fantastic for gut health because they get your heart pumping and your blood flowing, stimulating digestion. Activities like jogging, swimming, and cycling are excellent examples of cardio workouts. They help keep your digestive system active and running smoothly (Gastrointestinal Society, n.d.-a).
2. **Be consistent**: Any exercise is great, but regular exercise is far better. Just like eating a healthy diet, exercise consistency matters for gut health. Try incorporating physical activity into your daily routine to maintain a healthy gut over time (Boytar et al., 2023).
3. **Start small**: If you are new to exercise or have not been active for a while, it is perfectly okay to start with short walks, gentle stretches, or easy-paced activities. As you build your fitness level, you can gradually increase the intensity and duration of your workouts.
4. **Get outdoors**: Exercising outdoors has additional benefits. The fresh air and nature can reduce stress, which, as you already know, is good for your gut. So, whether it is a park, a beach, or just your backyard, consider taking your workouts outdoors whenever possible (Gladwell et al., 2013).

5. **Do not forget your nutrition**: Exercise and nutrition go hand in hand, so maintain a balanced diet to support your exercise routine as well as your gut health. Foods rich in fiber, like fruits, vegetables, and whole grains, can complement your exercise routine by promoting regular bowel movements and nourishing your gut microbiota.

OVERCOMING BARRIERS TO EXERCISE

Embarking on a journey to better health through exercise is commendable, but I appreciate that it can also be challenging. I would like to address some of the most common barriers to exercise and provide practical, actionable strategies for you to overcome them. My hope is that this will help you to achieve your fitness goals and maintain a healthy lifestyle.

I Have No Time!

Why not treat exercise like a necessary appointment and set specific times for workouts? Make them non-negotiable!

Prioritize shorter, more intense workouts like high-intensity interval training (HIIT), which can be efficient and effective while requiring less time.

My Friends and Family Do Not Share My Interest!

Why not find exercise buddies or join a group? Seek out friends or family members who might be interested in joining you for workouts.

Sign up for a local fitness class, club, or even an online community to connect with like-minded individuals who share your fitness goals.

I Just Do Not Have the Energy!

Why not set easily achievable targets? Break your fitness goals into smaller, more attainable milestones to stay motivated. Once you start exercising, you may well find you have more energy to spare.

Focus on how exercise makes you feel, not just on external factors such as weight loss. Find enjoyment in the process!

I Do Not Have Any Equipment!

Why not just use what you do have? Bodyweight exercises like push-ups, squats, and planks require no equipment and can be highly effective.

Be creative with household items. A chair can become a workout bench, and filled water bottles can serve as weights.

I Have Too Many Family Obligations!

Why not incorporate exercise into your family time? Plan family-friendly activities such as hiking, cycling, or playing active games together.

Look for local programs or classes that offer childcare services while you work out.

I Do Not Have Enough Self-Confidence!

Why not start with beginner-friendly workouts that match your current fitness level?

Track your progress and celebrate small achievements to gradually boost your confidence.

What if I Hurt Myself?

Why not start slow and learn the proper technique?

You can check with a fitness professional or trainer to ensure that you are using the correct form. Start with low-impact exercises and gradually progress to more challenging ones as your confidence and strength grow.

Ultimately, the key to overcoming these barriers is flexibility and adaptability. What works best for you may change over time, and that is to be expected. The most important thing is to keep moving and find ways to make physical activity a sustainable part of your life, no matter your obstacles.

In this chapter, we have looked at the advantages of physical activity for maintaining a healthy gut and learned practical tips for integrating more movement into your daily routine, laying a strong foundation for your overall well-being. In the next chapter, we will explore another powerful tool for enhancing your gut health: intermittent fasting.

7

HACK #6: GIVE IT A BREAK

INTERMITTENT FASTING FOR A HAPPY GUT

 "Fasting is the single greatest natural healing therapy. It is nature's ancient, universal 'remedy' for many problems."

— ELSON HAAS, MD, PREVENTIVE MEDICAL CENTER OF MARIN, USA

Have you ever wished you could press a reset button in life and give yourself a fresh start? Just as life occasionally calls for a reboot, our bodies may also benefit from a reset, particularly regarding our digestive system.

The demands of modern life can all too easily give you a perception of dwindling energy levels. You may feel fatigued and unable to think clearly, but your digestive health can also show signs of strain.

Let me introduce you to intermittent fasting—a practice that is like hitting the much-needed reset button for our digestive system, allowing it to rest and repair. In this chapter, we will explore the remarkable benefits of intermittent fasting for gut health and how it can be incorporated seamlessly into your daily routine.

THE PROBLEM WITH SNACKING AND LATE-NIGHT EATING

Snacking and late-night eating are not only bad for your waistline—they can also significantly impact your gut health, digestion, and overall well-being. Eating close to bedtime disrupts your natural digestive process, potentially leading to discomfort and indigestion and even affecting the quality of your sleep. Your body needs time to efficiently break down and absorb nutrients from your food (Leone et al., 2015).

Such eating habits can also have several other undesirable consequences, including the following:

1. **Weight gain**: Consistently eating excess calories in the late evening leads to gradual weight gain. During sleep, your body's energy expenditure is naturally lower, making it less effective at burning off the calories consumed late at night.
2. **Higher levels of fat in your blood**: Late-night snacking, especially on foods high in unhealthy fats or sugars, can result in elevated levels of harmful fats such as cholesterol and triglycerides in your bloodstream. These unhealthy fats can increase your risk of heart disease and metabolic disorders, negatively impacting your overall health.
3. **Increased hunger**: Late-night snacking may make you hungrier during waking hours. This can lead to overeating

and poor food choices throughout the day as you try to satisfy your heightened appetite.
4. **Slower energy usage**: Eating late at night can disrupt your body's natural patterns of energy usage. Instead of burning calories efficiently, your body may store them as fat, making it harder to maintain or lose weight.
5. **Circadian rhythm disruption**: Your body has an internal clock known as the circadian rhythm, which regulates various physiological processes including digestion. Late-night eating can disturb this rhythm, affecting hormone production and digestion and potentially leading to metabolic irregularities.
6. **Poorer sleep quality**: Eating food close to bedtime can disrupt your sleep quality. Digesting a large meal, spicy food, or high-sugar snacks can cause discomfort, heartburn, or indigestion, making it difficult to fall asleep and stay asleep throughout the night.

UNDERSTANDING INTERMITTENT FASTING

What Is Intermittent Fasting?

Intermittent fasting involves a special eating schedule. Instead of eating all day long, you have specific times for eating and specific times for fasting (i.e., not eating). It is not about what you eat but when you eat (Jaramillo et al., 2023).

Some popular approaches to intermittent fasting are the 16/8 method (fasting for 16 hours and eating for 8) and the 5:2 method (eating normally for five days of the week and eating small amounts for two days).

Why Should You Fast?

People try intermittent fasting for various reasons. One common goal is to lose weight. When you fast, your body uses its stored fat for energy, helping you to shed those extra pounds. It can also simplify your daily routine by reducing the meals you need to prepare and think about.

How Intermittent Fasting Affects Your Cells and Hormones

When you fast, your body adapts to the lower energy intake and becomes more efficient at burning fat. This includes a decrease in your levels of insulin, one of the hormones responsible for regulating your blood sugar, which can help with weight loss and reduce your risk of type 2 diabetes. Fasting also activates a very beneficial process called autophagy, where your cells clean out old and damaged cellular components.

Health Benefits

Intermittent fasting offers several other health benefits over and above weight loss. For instance, following this special eating pattern can improve your heart health by reducing risk factors such as cholesterol and blood pressure. It may also boost your brain function and help protect against age-related diseases.

Safety and Side Effects

Intermittent fasting is safe and well tolerated for most people. However, it is not suitable for everyone. Pregnant or breastfeeding women, children, and individuals with certain medical conditions should avoid it or consult a doctor first. In addition, some people may feel hungry, tired, or irritable during fasting periods, although these side effects often improve with time.

BENEFITS OF INTERMITTENT FASTING FOR GUT HEALTH

Intermittent fasting offers several significant benefits for your gut health. It promotes improved digestion and overall gut function, reduces inflammation and strengthens your immune system, and enhances the diversity and health of your gut microbiota. The changes in your gut microbiota that occur during intermittent fasting result from alterations in the gut environment, ultimately leading to a healthier digestive system (Hu et al., 2023). The details of these benefits are given below.

Improved Digestion and Gut Function

Intermittent fasting can significantly improve your digestion and overall gut function. When you give your gut scheduled breaks from having to digest food, it has the opportunity to rest and recuperate. This can enhance your digestive efficiency and improve the regularity of your bowel movements, contributing to better gut health.

Reduced Inflammation and Improved Immune Function

One important advantage of intermittent fasting is its potential to reduce inflammation within your gut. Chronic inflammation can disrupt your gut health and lead to various digestive issues. By practicing intermittent fasting, you can help mitigate this inflammation, thereby promoting a healthier gut lining. In addition, a healthier gut often goes hand in hand with a stronger immune system—a balanced gut can better defend against harmful pathogens, thus improving your overall immune function.

Enhanced Gut Microbiota Diversity and Health

Intermittent fasting can have a positive influence on your gut microbiota. It encourages the growth of beneficial microbes while inhibiting that of potentially harmful ones. As you will hopefully have learned while reading this book, a diverse and balanced microbiota is closely associated with better gut health and overall well-being.

Remodeling of the Gut Microbiota

The impact of intermittent fasting on the environment inside your gut can be advantageous for remodeling your gut microbiota. When you abstain from eating, less fuel and nutrients are available for the microbes living in your gut. This shift in available resources favors some microorganisms and disfavors others, which can be beneficial for gut health. Furthermore, intermittent fasting may increase the production of short-chain fatty acids, which serve as nutrition for the cells lining your colon. This can help maintain a healthy gut environment and contribute to a flourishing gut microbiota.

GETTING STARTED WITH INTERMITTENT FASTING

Intermittent fasting offers various approaches to structuring your eating habits, each with unique benefits and considerations. So let us explore some different types of intermittent fasting and learn clear instructions for each one, along with some common questions and answers that might benefit you.

Types of Intermittent Fasting

Time-Restricted Eating

Instructions: This method limits your daily eating to a specific time window, which is typically in the range of eight hours. For example, you might eat between 10 a.m. and 6 p.m. then fast for the remaining hours.

Question: Can I drink water or non-caloric beverages during the fasting period?

Answer: Yes, you are allowed to drink water, tea, or black coffee during the fasting period, as long as they do not contain added calories.

Question: Is it okay to exercise during the fasting period?

Answer: Yes, it is generally safe to exercise during your fasting hours. However, some people may find exercising more comfortable during the eating window.

Question: What can I eat during the eating window?

Answer: You should eat a balanced diet during your eating window. As we discussed in Chapters 3 and 4, focus on whole foods, lean proteins, fruits, vegetables, and whole grains.

The 5:2 Method

Instructions: In this approach, you eat normally for five days of the week and restrict your calorie intake to around 500–600 calories on the other two non-consecutive days. For example, you may choose to fast on Tuesday and Friday and eat normally for the rest of the week.

Question: Can I choose any two days for the low-calorie intake?

Answer: Yes, you can select any two days that work best for your schedule, as long as they are not consecutive days.

Alternate-Day Fasting

Instructions: This method involves alternating between fasting days, when you consume very few calories or none at all, and regular eating days.

Question: Can I drink beverages with calories on fasting days?

Answer: Sticking to non-caloric beverages on fasting days is recommended to maximize the benefits.

The 24-Hour Fast

Instructions: With this method, you fast for a full 24 hours once or twice a week, abstaining from all food and calorie-containing beverages. It is also called the "eat stop eat" method.

Question: Should I do this type of fasting more than twice a week?

Answer: It is generally recommended to start with once or twice a week and consult a healthcare professional if you are considering doing it more frequently.

Which Intermittent Fasting Schedule Is Best?

The best intermittent fasting schedule is the one that aligns with your lifestyle and is sustainable for your needs. Each person is different, so it is crucial to choose a method that you can adhere to in the long term. Feel free to experiment!

The Importance of Consulting a Doctor

Before starting any type of diet, including intermittent fasting, it is advisable to consult with your healthcare provider, especially if you suffer from underlying health conditions or are taking medications.

Frequently Asked Questions

Is Intermittent Fasting Safe for Everyone?

Intermittent fasting may not be suitable for pregnant or breast-feeding women, children, individuals with eating disorders, or those with certain medical conditions. It is advisable to consult with your doctor before starting.

Can I Drink Water During Fasting Hours?

Yes, staying hydrated with water is encouraged during your fasting hours.

Will Intermittent Fasting Slow Down My Metabolism?

When done correctly, intermittent fasting typically does not significantly slow down your metabolism. In fact, it can support weight management.

Can I Continue My Regular Exercise Routine During Intermittent Fasting?

Yes, you can exercise during fasting hours, but listen to your body and adjust your routine as needed.

What Should I Eat During the Eating Window?

You should focus on a balanced diet based on whole foods, including lean proteins, fruits, vegetables, and whole grains.

How Long Does It Take to See Results?

Results vary among individuals, but some people may notice changes in their weight and overall well-being within just a few weeks. Remember that each person's experience with intermittent fasting may differ, so monitoring your health and consulting a healthcare professional for personalized guidance is essential.

How Can I Suppress Hunger During Intermittent Fasting?

Managing your hunger during intermittent fasting can be achieved by staying hydrated with water, herbal tea, or black coffee during your fasting hours. Consuming high-fiber foods, lean proteins, and healthy fats during your eating windows can also help keep you feel full.

When Should I Exercise?

The ideal time to exercise during intermittent fasting may vary between individuals. Some people prefer to work out during their fasting hours to maximize fat burning, while others find exercising more comfortable during their eating windows. Choose a time that suits your energy levels and schedule.

Is It Okay to Skip Breakfast?

Yes, skipping breakfast is common in many intermittent fasting schedules, such as the 16/8 method. The focus is on when you eat, not necessarily when breakfast traditionally occurs.

How Do I Combat Feelings of Low Energy or Low Focus?

To combat low energy or low focus, prioritize nutritious meals during your eating windows, including complex carbohydrates, proteins, and healthy fats. Staying hydrated and incorporating electrolytes can also help you maintain your energy levels. Gradually adapting to intermittent fasting can reduce these symptoms over time.

Can I Drink Alcohol?

Consuming alcohol during intermittent fasting should be done cautiously. Alcohol can affect your blood sugar levels and may interfere with the fasting state. If you do choose to drink alcohol, do so in moderation and consider aligning it with your eating window.

Does Fasting Benefit People Who Do Not Need to Lose Weight?

Yes, intermittent fasting also offers benefits beyond weight loss. It can improve your metabolic health, support cognitive function, enhance energy levels, and promote longevity. People with a healthy weight or specific health goals can still find value in intermittent fasting for their overall well-being.

SETTING YOURSELF UP FOR INTERMITTENT FASTING SUCCESS

The following six points should help you on your journey to intermittent fasting success:

1. **Take it slowly**: Start gradually. Do not immediately jump into a strict fasting regimen. Extend your fasting window by an hour or two at a time, gradually increasing it as your body becomes accustomed to the new routine.
2. **Choose the plan that suits you best**: Try to select a regimen that aligns with your daily routine and preferences. If you have a busy schedule, consider a plan that suits your lifestyle, such as the 16/8 method. Flexibility is the key to long-term success.
3. **Avoid overeating during your eating windows**: Pay attention to your portion sizes and food quality. Overindulging during your eating windows can negate the benefits of fasting. Focus on balanced, nutrient-dense meals that satisfy you without excessive calorie intake.
4. **Eat enough to meet your body's nutritional needs**: Ensure that you consume sufficient calories and nutrients

to support your energy needs and overall health. Restricting your calories excessively during your eating windows can lead to nutrient deficiencies and low energy levels.
5. **Focus on diet quality as well as when you eat**: While meal timing is an important aspect of intermittent fasting, do not disregard the quality of your food. Prioritize a well-rounded diet rich in whole foods, including lean proteins, fruits, vegetables, and whole grains.
6. **Stay hydrated**: Hydration is crucial. Drink water, herbal tea, or black coffee during your fasting hours to stay hydrated and help control your hunger. However, pay attention to your caffeine intake to avoid dehydration.

By taking these precautions and being mindful of your body's needs, you can set yourself up for success in intermittent fasting. Remember that your intermittent fasting regimen should be sustainable and tailored to your individual lifestyle and goals.

It is important to remember that everyone's journey with intermittent fasting is unique. Your experience may differ from that of your friend or the person you follow on social media. That is perfectly okay! It is crucial to tailor your approach to your own personal needs. The beauty of intermittent fasting is its flexibility. However, if you have specific health concerns or dietary requirements, consulting your healthcare provider is always a good idea. They can offer personalized guidance and ensure that you are on the right track to a healthier you.

In this chapter, we have examined the world of intermittent fasting, discussing its significant impact on gut health while shedding light on the various approaches and potential pitfalls to watch out for.

In the final chapter of our journey, we will examine another vital aspect of gut health—dietary supplements such as probiotics. We will consider the advantages of these products and help you choose high-quality options that align with your goals for improving your gut health.

HACK #7: FUEL UP

SUPPLEMENTING YOUR GUT

> *"I don't think anybody needs supplements but only under certain conditions: (1) you have to hunt and gather your own wild food, (2) you have to drink pure clean water, (3) you have to have no chronic stress, (4) you have to exercise all the time as part of your lifestyle, (5) you have to sleep nine hours a night going to bed with the sun and waking with the sun, and (6) you have to be exposed to no environmental toxins or external insults. Now if that's you, no, you don't need any supplements, but the rest of us, we should pay attention!"*
>
> — MARK HYMAN, MD, THE ULTRAWELLNESS CENTER, USA

In an ideal world, we should obtain all of our essential nutrients from whole foods. However, life can throw curveballs, and all of us may sometimes need extra support for our gut health. This is where nutritional supplements such as probiotics come into play (Hyman, 2022).

This last chapter is about uncovering the valuable benefits of supplements for nurturing your gut health. We will examine how these products can provide that much-needed boost and enhance your overall well-being. However, not all supplements are created equal. There is a vast array of options, and choosing the right product can make all the difference. That is why a significant portion of this chapter is dedicated to providing practical guidance on selecting a high-quality product that aligns with your gut health goals.

While whole foods remain the gold standard, let us embrace the potential of supplements such as probiotics as valuable allies in our quest for optimal gut health. This chapter is your roadmap to understanding their benefits and making informed choices. So let us get started on the path to a healthier gut!

OVERVIEW OF DIETARY SUPPLEMENTS

You must understand the basics of dietary supplements to make an informed choice when standing in the supplement aisle of your local pharmacy facing hundreds of different products. So what are dietary supplements, what can they do for you, and how do you choose the best one?

What Are Dietary Supplements?

Dietary supplements are products intended to provide additional nutrients that may be absent from or not present in sufficient amounts in a person's regular diet. They come in various forms, including vitamins, minerals, herbs, botanicals, amino acids (the building blocks of proteins), enzymes, and other substances (Incze, 2019).

What Are the Benefits of Dietary Supplements?

The potential advantages of taking dietary supplements vary depending on the specific supplement and the individual's health needs. Some possible benefits include the following:

- **Higher intake of specific nutrients**: Dietary supplements can help fill nutrient gaps in your diet, ensuring that you get the vitamins and minerals your body needs for various functions.
- **Support for specific health conditions**: Some supplements are designed to address specific health problems or support certain aspects of your well-being. For example, calcium and vitamin D supplements can support bone health, while omega-3 fatty acids may promote heart health.
- **Convenience**: Supplements can be an easy way to obtain essential nutrients, especially for individuals with dietary restrictions or busy lifestyles.
- **Targeted fitness goals**: Athletes, bodybuilders, and people with specific fitness goals may use supplements such as protein powders, creatine, or branched-chain amino acids to aid muscle growth, recovery, and performance.

What Are the Risks of Dietary Supplements?

Although dietary supplements can offer benefits, there are also potential risks and considerations to keep in mind, including the following (Ronis et al., 2018):

- **Safety concerns**: Unfortunately, not all dietary supplements are rigorously tested for safety and efficacy before being put on the market. The quality and potential risks can vary, but some products may lead to potential adverse effects.
- **Drug-nutrient interactions**: Some supplements can interact with medications or other supplements, potentially causing unwanted side effects or reducing the effectiveness of the medication.
- **Overconsumption**: Excessive intake of specific vitamins and minerals through supplements can lead to harmful health effects. It is essential to follow the recommended dosages.
- **Lack of regulation**: The regulation of dietary supplements varies by country, and some products may not be subjected to the same extensive testing and quality control procedures as pharmaceutical drugs.
- **Not a replacement for a balanced diet**: Dietary supplements are intended to complement a healthy diet, not replace it. Relying solely on supplements, therefore, can lead to nutrient imbalances or other health problems.

CHOOSING A SUPPLEMENT TO SUPPORT YOUR GUT HEALTH

What Do Gut Health Supplements Do?

As the name suggests, gut health supplements are designed to target various aspects of your digestive system, which we have already learned can promote your overall well-being. Here are some examples of ways that supplements can promote your gut health:

- **Digestion**: Some supplements are intended to improve the breakdown of food and absorption of nutrients, ensuring your body gets the most from your food.
- **Microbiota balance**: Some supplements aim to support a balanced and diverse gut microbiota, which is essential for your overall health.
- **Regularity**: Some supplements help regulate your bowel movements, preventing constipation or diarrhea.
- **Digestive comfort**: Some supplements can ease discomfort caused by indigestion, bloating, or gas.

Common Gut Health Supplements

Some of the most common types of gut health supplements are listed below:

1. **Probiotics**: Probiotic supplements contain live microorganisms intended to promote and maintain a healthy gut microbiota. Products containing various species and strains of beneficial microbes are available, each with unique benefits (Youssef et al., 2021).
2. **Digestive enzymes**: These enzymes assist in breaking down food, making nutrients more accessible for absorption (Ianiro et al., 2016).
3. **Bacteriophages**: These target and eliminate harmful bacteria in the gut, supporting a balanced microbiota (Kiani et al., 2020).
4. **Prebiotics**: Prebiotics contain soluble dietary fiber, which serves as food for the good microbes in your gut (Davani-Davari et al., 2019).
5. **Psyllium**: Psyllium fiber can promote regular bowel movements and relieve constipation (Jalanka et al., 2019).

6. **Vitamin C**: This antioxidant supports gut health and overall immunity (Hazan et al., 2022).
7. **Zinc L-carnosine**: This supplement can help protect the gut lining and support digestive comfort (Mahmood et al., 2007).
8. **L-Glutamine**: L-Glutamine is a naturally occurring amino acid that aids in repairing the gut lining (Perna et al., 2019).
9. **Licorice**: Licorice root can help soothe digestive discomfort and inflammation (Bethapudi et al., 2022).
10. **Curcumin**: This anti-inflammatory compound found in turmeric may benefit gut health by reducing inflammation (Scazzocchio et al., 2020).

TIPS FOR INCORPORATING SUPPLEMENTS IN YOUR DAILY LIFE

It is essential to get the most out of your supplements in order to maintain your overall health. To maximize the benefits of your supplement regimen, consider the following tips:

1. **Create a plan**: Before starting to take supplements, it is crucial to have a clear plan in place. Identify your specific health goals and nutritional needs to determine which supplements are right for you. A well-considered plan will keep you focused and motivated.
2. **Follow instructions**: Always adhere to the recommended dosage and instructions provided on the supplement label or suggested by your healthcare provider. Taking more than the recommended dose can be harmful and may not offer additional benefits.
3. **Consider timing**: The timing of supplement intake can influence effectiveness. Some supplements are best taken with food to enhance absorption, whereas others are more

effective on an empty stomach. Tailor the timing to your specific supplements and individual needs, and consider any potential interactions with other medications that you are taking.

4. **Create a routine**: Make taking your supplements a part of your daily routine. Consistency is vital, so find a time that works for you, whether that means with your morning coffee or before bedtime, and stick to it.
5. **Get organized**: Consider using a pill organizer or setting reminders on your phone to avoid confusion and missed doses. Keep your supplements in a convenient and visible location to ensure you remember to take them. Note that some supplement containers are specifically designed to maintain the integrity of the supplements they contain, so using a pill organizer is not always recommended. Probiotics, for example, usually require a controlled environment to ensure that the living microorganisms remain viable.
6. **Be patient**: Understand that supplements may take time to show noticeable effects. Being patient is crucial, as the impact on your health can be gradual and individual responses may vary.
7. **Choose quality supplements**: Select supplements from reputable brands that adhere to good manufacturing practices. High-quality supplements are more likely to contain the stated ingredients in the right amounts and without harmful contaminants.

Gut health supplements can kickstart the well-being of your gut microbiota and digestive tract. Not everyone will benefit from taking supplements, however, and they can be an expensive option that stretches your monthly budget.

A healthy, well-balanced, whole-food diet is the cornerstone of your overall health and wellness. Supplements are designed to support your diet, enabling you to reach your health goals sooner. In other words, they should not be used in place of a nutritious diet. Not only will they be less effective, but they will also not improve your gut health over the long term.

KEEPING THE GAME ALIVE

Now that you have everything you need to make peace with food, achieve mental clarity, and improve your overall health from the inside out, it's time to share your knowledge and guide others to the same help.

If you enjoyed my book, I'd love to hear your thoughts—please consider leaving a review on whichever platform you purchased it from! You'll show other readers where they can find the information they're seeking and help spread the word about gut health.

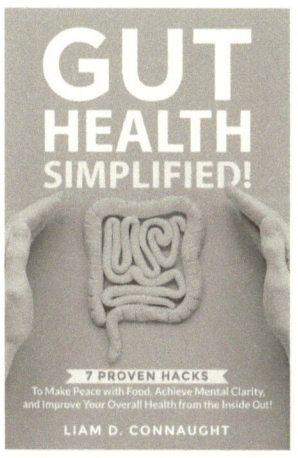

Thank you for your help. Gut health is kept alive when we share what we've learned—and you're helping me do just that.

Stay connected and join the conversation—visit our Facebook and Instagram pages *Gut Health Simplified* for updates, discussions, and more!

CONCLUSION

 "A healthy gut is the gateway to a healthy body and mind."

— MARK HYMAN, MD, THE ULTRAWELLNESS CENTER, USA

These words encapsulate the essence of our exploration into gut health—a healthy gut is the foundation upon which a healthy body and mind are built.

My sincere hope is that this book has provided a comprehensive and holistic approach to enhancing your gut health and overall well-being.

Throughout this book, I have sought to present systematic and practical strategies to address the underlying causes of gut-related issues, with the ultimate goal of helping you achieve profound improvements in your health.

I hope that your journey through these pages has been enlightening and helped you uncover the intricate world of your gut health. I have attempted to dismantle the complex science behind the topics discussed and offer a clear and accessible understanding of the simple principles that can empower you to achieve optimal wellness.

I have also emphasized the pivotal roles that factors such as diet, stress, and lifestyle choices play in shaping the state of your gut and, by extension, your overall health. However, while the scientific aspects of gut health are intriguing, the real-life transformations testify to the importance of prioritizing this facet of your well-being.

You have seen how implementing my seven hacks could lead to remarkable changes in your life. From improved digestion to increased energy levels, mental clarity to reduced stress and anxiety, better sleep to an enhanced immune system, and ultimately an overall better quality of life—these tangible rewards await those prioritizing their gut health.

These transformative principles have the potential to guide you toward a happier and healthier gut, which, in turn, can significantly impact your overall well-being.

As we conclude this enlightening journey, I urge you to turn your newfound knowledge into concrete actions. Embrace the seven hacks for a happy gut and integrate them into your daily routine. Recognize that even the smallest changes can yield substantial improvements in your health, as long as they are maintained consistently. The journey to optimal gut health begins with this commitment, and your digestive system will undoubtedly thank you.

If you have found value in this book and it has led you to experience positive changes in your life, I humbly request your review. Your feedback can serve as a beacon of inspiration for others embarking on their own path to a healthier gut and an improved quality of life. Together, we can create a vibrant community of empowered individuals committed to their health, extending the ripple effect of wellness far beyond the confines of these pages and into the lives of countless others.

It is crucial to remember that your health is your most valuable asset. By prioritizing your gut health, you are taking a significant step toward a brighter and healthier future. Embrace these principles, trust in your body's inherent wisdom, and nurture the extraordinary potential within you. The journey to improved gut health starts today, offering you a path to well-being that will empower you for a lifetime.

As you embark on this journey, let me leave you with a powerful reminder: You are the architect of your own health.

Your body has an innate ability to heal and thrive when provided with the right tools and knowledge. Just like a skilled craftsman meticulously builds a masterpiece, you can create your own masterpiece of health and well-being. Every choice you make, whether that means the food you put on your plate or how you manage stress, shapes your gut health and overall vitality. It is within your power to make these choices wisely and intentionally. As you do, you will be crafting a life filled with boundless energy, mental clarity, and a sense of well-being that radiates from within.

Think of your journey to better gut health as laying the foundation for a beautiful and enduring structure. Each choice you make, each step you take, is like a carefully placed brick reinforcing the strength and stability of your foundation. Over time, your efforts will build a robust and resilient structure that supports a life of health, vibrancy, and fulfillment.

Improving your gut health is not a destination but rather an ongoing journey. It is a commitment to yourself and a dedication to nurturing your body and mind with the care and attention they deserve.

Along this journey, you may encounter challenges, setbacks, and moments of doubt, but these are all part of the process. They are the stones you encounter on the path, each offering an opportunity for growth and resilience.

So, as you start, remember that every decision you make is a step toward greater well-being. Your body is an incredible and intricate masterpiece, and you have the brush in your hand to paint a vibrant and healthy life. Embrace this opportunity, trust in the wisdom of your body, and keep moving forward, one choice at a time.

Your health is a lifelong endeavor, and improving your gut health is one of the most profound and rewarding steps you can take. It is a gift to yourself, an investment in your future, and a declaration that you value life's vitality and your own well-being. So, take the first step toward improving your gut health today, and let this journey be a testament to your commitment to a life of health, happiness, and fulfillment. Your gut will thank you, and your future self will be grateful for your choices to prioritize your health and well-being.

REFERENCES

NOTE: The sources listed below are intended as further reading if you wish to examine in more detail some of the key points made in the part of the text they are cited, as researched and discussed in the medical and scientific arena.

Ahmad, R. (2015, May 20). *How Much Water Do You Need Each Day?* Penn Medicine, Retrieved January 27, 2024, https://www.pennmedicine.org/updates/blogs/health-and-wellness/2015/may/how-much-water-do-you-need-each-day

Albuquerque, T. G., Bragotto, A. P. A., & Costa, H. S. (2022). Processed Food: Nutrition, Safety, and Public Health. *International Journal of Environmental Research and Public Health, 19*(24), Article 16410. https://doi.org/10.3390/ijerph192416410

American Psychological Association. (2019, October 30). *Mindfulness Meditation: A Research-Proven Way to Reduce Stress.* American Psychological Association. Retrieved January 27, 2024, https://www.apa.org/topics/mindfulness/meditation

Aslam, H., Marx, W., Rocks, T., Loughman, A., Chandrasekaran, V., Ruusunen, A., Dawson, S. L., West, M., Mullarkey, E., Pasco, J. A., & Jacka, F. N. (2020). The effects of dairy and dairy derivatives on the gut microbiota: a systematic literature review. *Gut Microbes, 12*(1), Article 1799533. https://doi.org/10.1080/19490976.2020.1799533

Bansal, S., Connolly, M., & Harder, T. (2021). Impact of a Whole-Foods, Plant-Based Nutrition Intervention on Patients Living with Chronic Disease in an Underserved Community. *American Journal of Lifestyle Medicine, 16*(3), 382–389. https://doi.org/10.1177/15598276211018159

Banskota, S., Ghia, J.-E., & Khan, W. I. (2019). Serotonin in the gut: Blessing or a curse. *Biochimie, 161,* 56–64. https://doi.org/10.1016/j.biochi.2018.06.008

Barber, T. M., Kabisch, S., Pfeiffer, A. F. H., & Weickert, M. O. (2020). The Health Benefits of Dietary Fibre. *Nutrients, 12*(10), Article 3209. https://doi.org/10.3390/nu12103209

Belobrajdic, D. P., James-Martin, G., Jones, D., & Tran, C. D. (2023). Soy and Gastrointestinal Health: A Review. *Nutrients, 15*(8), Article 1959. https://doi.org/10.3390/nu15081959

Benincasa, P., Falcinelli, B., Lutts, S., Stagnari, F., & Galieni, A. (2019). Sprouted Grains: A Comprehensive Review. *Nutrients, 11*(2), Article 421. https://doi.org/10.3390/nu11020421

Bethapudi, B., Murugan, S. K., Nithyanantham, M., Singh, V., Agarwal, A., & Mundkinajeddu, D. (2022). Gut health benefits of licorice and its flavonoids as dietary supplements. *Nutrition and Functional Foods in Boosting Digestion, Metabolism and Immune Health*, 377–417. https://doi.org/10.1016/b978-0-12-821232-5.00008-2

Borkoles, E., Krastins, D., van der Pols, J. C., Sims, P., & Polman, R. (2022). Short-Term Effect of Additional Daily Dietary Fibre Intake on Appetite, Satiety, Gastrointestinal Comfort, Acceptability, and Feasibility. *Nutrients, 14*(19), Article 4214. https://doi.org/10.3390/nu14194214

Boytar, A. N., Skinner, T. L., Wallen, R. E., Jenkins, D. G., & Dekker Nitert, M. (2023). The Effect of Exercise Prescription on the Human Gut Microbiota and Comparison between Clinical and Apparently Healthy Populations: A Systematic Review. *Nutrients, 15*(6), Article 1534. https://doi.org/10.3390/nu15061534

Carter, K. S., & Carter, R. C., III (2016). Breath-based meditation: A mechanism to restore the physiological and cognitive reserves for optimal human performance. *World Journal of Clinical Cases, 4*(4), 99-102. https://doi.org/10.12998/wjcc.v4.i4.99

Centers for Disease Control and Prevention. (2022, September 8). *Poor Nutrition.* Retrieved January 27, 2024, https://www.cdc.gov/chronicdisease/resources/publications/factsheets/nutrition.htm

Chang, L. (2011). The Role of Stress on Physiologic Responses and Clinical Symptoms in Irritable Bowel Syndrome. *Gastroenterology, 140*(3), 761-765.E5. https://doi.org/10.1053/j.gastro.2011.01.032

Chattu, V., Manzar, M. D., Kumary, S., Burman, D., Spence, D., & Pandi-Perumal, S. R. (2019). The Global Problem of Insufficient Sleep and Its Serious Public Health Implications. *Healthcare, 7*(1), Article 7010001. https://doi.org/10.3390/healthcare7010001

Chow, C. M. (2022). Sleep Hygiene Practices: Where to Now? *Hygiene, 2*(3), 146–151. https://doi.org/10.3390/hygiene2030013

Christian, B. (2022, March 14). *So, You Want to Increase your Fiber Intake?* UMass Chan Medical School. Retrieved January 24, 2024, https://www.umassmed.edu/nutrition/blog/blog-posts/2022/3/so-you-want-to-increase-your-fiber-intake

Cleveland Clinic. (2022, January 31). *How to Practice Mindful Eating.* Cleveland Clinic. Retrieved January 24, 2024, https://health.clevelandclinic.org/mindful-eating

Complete Pilates. (n.d.-a). *Criss Cross Exercise - Your Step by Step Guide with Video!* Complete Pilates. Retrieved January 24, 2024, https://complete-pilates.co.uk/criss-cross-exercise

Complete Pilates (n.d.-b). *How to avoid back pain with the swan exercise.* Complete Pilates. Retrieved January 24, 2024, https://complete-pilates.co.uk/pilates-swan

Complete Pilates. (n.d.-c). *Pelvic Clock- Your Step by Step Guide with Video!* Complete

Pilates. Retrieved January 24, 2024, https://complete-pilates.co.uk/pelvic-clock

Convertino, V. A., Armstrong, L. E., Coyle, E. F., Mack, G. W., Sawka, M. N., Senay, L. C., & Sherman, W. M. (1996). ACSM Position Stand: Exercise and Fluid Replacement. *Medicine & Science in Sports & Exercise, 28*(10), i–ix. https://doi.org/10.1097/00005768-199610000-00045

Davani-Davari, D., Negahdaripour, M., Karimzadeh, I., Seifan, M., Mohkam, M., Masoumi, S., Berenjian, A., & Ghasemi, Y. (2019). Prebiotics: Definition, Types, Sources, Mechanisms, and Clinical Applications. *Foods, 8*(3), Article 92. https://doi: 10.3390/foods8030092

Dibay Moghadam, S., Krieger, J. W., & Louden, D. K. N. (2020). A Systematic Review of the Effectiveness of Promoting Water Intake to Reduce Sugar-sweetened Beverage Consumption. *Obesity Science & Practice, 6*(3), 229–246. https://doi.org/10.1002/osp4.397

El-Sharkawy, A. M., Sahota, O., & Lobo, D. N. (2015). Acute and Chronic Effects of Hydration Status on Health. *Nutrition Reviews, 73*(2), 97–109. https://doi.org/10.1093/nutrit/nuv038

Fernández-Castañeda, A., Lu, P., Geraghty, A. C., Song, E., Lee, M.-H., Wood, J., O'Dea, M. R., Dutton, S., Shamardani, K., Nwangwu, K., Mancusi, R., Yalçın, B., Taylor, K. R., Acosta-Alvarez, L., Malacon, K., Keough, M. B., Ni, L., Woo, P. J., Contreras-Esquivel, D., & Toland, A. M. S. (2022). Mild respiratory COVID can cause multi-lineage neural cell and myelin dysregulation. *Cell, 185*(14), 2452-2468.e16. https://doi.org/10.1016/j.cell.2022.06.008

Foster, J. A., Rinaman, L., & Cryan, J. F. (2017). Stress & the gut-brain axis: Regulation by the microbiome. *Neurobiology of Stress, 7,* 124–136. https://doi.org/10.1016/j.ynstr.2017.03.001

Fryar, C. D., Carroll, M. D., & Afful, J. (2020). *Prevalence of Overweight, Obesity, and Extreme Obesity Among Adults Aged 20 and Over: United States, 1960–1962 Through 2017–2018.* National Center for Health Statistics. Retrieved January 27, 2024, https://www.cdc.gov/nchs/data/hestat/obesity-adult-17-18/obesity-adult.htm

Gao, F., Guo, R., Ma, Q., Li, Y., Wang, W., Fan, Y., Ju, Y., Zhao, B., Gao, Y., Qian, L., Yang, Z., He, X., Jin, X., Liu, Y., Peng, Y., Chen, C., Chen, Y., Gao, C., Zhu, F., & Ma, X. (2022). Stressful events induce long-term gut microbiota dysbiosis and associated post-traumatic stress symptoms in healthcare workers fighting against COVID-19. *Journal of Affective Disorders, 303,* 187–195. https://doi.org/10.1016/j.jad.2022.02.024

Garcia, K., Ferreira, G., Reis, F., & Viana, S. (2022). Impact of Dietary Sugars on Gut Microbiota and Metabolic Health. *Diabetology, 3*(4), 549–560. https://doi.org/10.3390/diabetology3040042

Garcia-Mazcorro, J. F., Noratto, G., & Remes-Troche, J. M. (2018). The Effect of Gluten-Free Diet on Health and the Gut Microbiota Cannot Be Extrapolated from One Population to Others. *Nutrients, 10*(10), Article 1421. https://doi.org/10.3390/nu10101421

Gastrointestinal Society. (n.d.-a). *Physical Activity and GI Health.* Gastrointestinal Society, Canadian Society of Intestinal Research. Retrieved January 27, 2024, https://badgut.org/information-centre/a-z-digestive-topics/physical-activity-and-gi-health

Gastrointestinal Society. (n.d.-b). *Stress Management,* Gastrointestinal Society, Canadian Society of Intestinal Research. Retrieved January 27, 2024, https://badgut.org/information-centre/a-z-digestive-topics/stress-management

Ge, L., Liu, S., Li, S., Yang, J., Hu, G., Xu, C., & Song, W. (2022). Psychological stress in inflammatory bowel disease: Psychoneuroimmunological insights into bidirectional gut-brain communications. *Frontiers in Immunology, 13,* Article 1016578. https://doi.org/10.3389/fimmu.2022.1016578

Gladwell, V. F., Brown, D. K., Wood, C., Sandercock, G. R., & Barton, J. L. (2013). The great outdoors: how a green exercise environment can benefit all. *Extreme Physiology & Medicine 2,* 3. https://doi.org/10.1186/2046-7648-2-3

Greger, M. (2020). A Whole Food Plant-Based Diet Is Effective for Weight Loss: The Evidence. *American Journal of Lifestyle Medicine, 14*(5), 500–510. https://doi.org/10.1177/1559827620912400

Grillo, A., Salvi, L., Coruzzi, P., Salvi, P., & Parati, G. (2019). Sodium Intake and Hypertension. *Nutrients, 11*(9), Article 1970. https://doi.org/10.3390/nu11091970

Gutierrez, E., Metcalfe, J. J., & Prescott, M. P. (2022). The Relationship between Fluid Milk, Water, and 100% Juice and Health Outcomes among Children and Adolescents. *Nutrients, 14*(9), Article 1892. https://doi.org/10.3390/nu14091892

Hadadi, N., Berweiler, V., Wang, H., & Trajkovski, M. (2021). Intestinal microbiota as a route for micronutrient bioavailability. *Current Opinion in Endocrine and Metabolic Research, 20,* Article 100285. https://doi.org/10.1016/j.coemr.2021.100285

Han, Y., & Xiao, H. (2020). Whole Food-Based Approaches to Modulating Gut Microbiota and Associated Diseases. *Annual Review of Food Science and Technology, 11,* 119–143. https://doi.org/10.1146/annurev-food-111519-014337

Harkins, P., Burke, E., Swales, C., & Silman, A. (2021). "All disease begins in the gut" —the role of the intestinal microbiome in ankylosing spondylitis. *Rheumatology Advances in Practice, 5*(3), Article rkab063. https://doi.org/10.1093/rap/rkab063

Harvard Health. (2016a, January 16). *8 steps to mindful eating.* Harvard Health Publishing - Harvard Medical School. Retrieved January 24, 2024, https://www.health.harvard.edu/staying-healthy/8-steps-to-mindful-eating

Harvard Health. (2016b, March 10). *Learning diaphragmatic breathing.* Harvard

Health Publishing - Harvard Medical School. Retrieved January 24, 2024, https://www.health.harvard.edu/healthbeat/learning-diaphragmatic-breathing

Harvard T.H. Chan School of Public Health. (n.d.). *Water*. The Nutrition Source; Harvard T.H. Chan School of Public Health. Retrieved January 24, 2024, https://www.hsph.harvard.edu/nutritionsource/water

Hasan, N., & Yang, H. (2019). Factors affecting the composition of the gut microbiota, and its modulation. *PeerJ*, 7, Article e7502. https://doi.org/10.7717/peerj.7502

Hazan, S., Dave, S., Papoutsis, A. J., Deshpande, N., Howell, M. C., & Martin, L. M. (2022). Vitamin C improves gut Bifidobacteria in humans. *Future Microbiology*. https://doi.org/10.2217/fmb-2022-0209

Henry Ford Health. (2021, July 26). *How Stress Affects Digestion—And What You Can Do About It*. Henry Ford Health. Retrieved January 24, 2024, https://www.henryford.com/blog/2021/07/how-stress-affects-digestion

Hu, X., Xia, K., Dai, M., Han, X., Yuan, P., Liu, J., Liu, S., Jia, F., Chen, J., Jiang, F., Yu, J., Yang, H., Wang, J., Xu, X., Jin, X., Kristiansen, K., Xiao, L., Chen, W., Han, M., & Duan, S. (2023). Intermittent fasting modulates the intestinal microbiota and improves obesity and host energy metabolism. *Npj Biofilms and Microbiomes*, 9, 19. https://doi.org/10.1038/s41522-023-00386-4

Hyman, M. (2022, April 18). *The 3 Daily Supplements Everyone Should Be Taking For Longevity: The Doctor's Farmacy with Mark Hyman M.D. #218* [Video]. YouTube. https://www.youtube.com/watch?v=6w0uvlWwEOk

Ianiro, G., Pecere, S., Giorgio, V., Gasbarrini, A., & Cammarota, G. (2016). Digestive Enzyme Supplementation in Gastrointestinal Diseases. *Current Drug Metabolism*, 17(2), 187–193. https://doi.org/10.2174/1389200217021601141501377

Incze, M. (2019). Vitamins and Nutritional Supplements. *JAMA Internal Medicine*, 179(3), 460. https://doi.org/10.1001/jamainternmed.2018.5880

Isaak, C. K., & Siow, Y. L. (2013). The evolution of nutrition research. *Canadian Journal of Physiology and Pharmacology*, 91(4), 257–267. https://doi.org/10.1139/cjpp-2012-0367

Jalanka, J., Major, G., Murray, K., Singh, G., Nowak, A., Kurtz, C., Silos-Santiago, I., Johnston, J., de Vos, W., & Spiller, R. (2019). The Effect of Psyllium Husk on Intestinal Microbiota in Constipated Patients and Healthy Controls. *International Journal of Molecular Sciences*, 20(2), Article 433. https://doi.org/10.3390/ijms20020433

Jaramillo, A., Castells, J., Ibrahimli, S., Jaramillo, L., Briones, R. R., Moncada, D., & Revilla, J. C. (2023). Time-Restricted Feeding and Intermittent Fasting as Preventive Therapeutics: A Systematic Review of the Literature. *Cureus*, 15(7), Article e42300. https://doi.org/10.7759/cureus.42300

Jones, J. M., García, C. G., & Braun, H. J. (2020). Perspective: Whole and Refined

Grains and Health—Evidence Supporting "Make Half Your Grains Whole." *Advances in Nutrition, 11*(3). 492-506. https://doi.org/10.1093/advances/nmz114

Kiani, A. K., Anpilogov, K., Dautaj, A., Marceddu, G., Sonna, W. N., Percio, M., Dundar, M., Beccari, T., & Bertelli, M. (2020). Bacteriophages in food supplements obtained from natural sources. *Acta Biomedica 91*(13-S), Article e2020025. https://doi.org/10.23750/abm.v91i13-S.10834

Killer, S. C., Blannin, A. K., & Jeukendrup, A. E. (2014). No Evidence of Dehydration with Moderate Daily Coffee Intake: A Counterbalanced Cross-Over Study in a Free-Living Population. *PLoS ONE, 9*(1), Article e84154. https://doi.org/10.1371/journal.pone.0084154

Koob, G. F. (2019, December 1). *It's holiday party season – here's what you need to know about the science of hangovers.* National Institute on Alcohol Abuse and Alcoholism (NIAAA). Retrieved January 26, 2024, https://www.niaaa.nih.gov/about-niaaa/directors-page/niaaa-directors-blog/its-holiday-party-season-heres-what-you-need-know-about-science-hangovers

Kruis, W., Forstmaier, G., Scheurlen, C., & Stellaard, F. (1991). Effect of diets low and high in refined sugars on gut transit, bile acid metabolism, and bacterial fermentation. *Gut 32*(4), 367–371. https://doi.org/10.1136/gut.32.4.367

Lattimer, J. M., & Haub, M. D. (2010). Effects of Dietary Fiber and Its Components on Metabolic Health. *Nutrients, 2*(12), 1266–1289. https://doi.org/10.3390/nu2121266

Lee, S. H., Moore, L.V., Park, S., Harris, D.M., Blanck H.M., (2022). Adults Meeting Fruit and Vegetable Intake Recommendations — United States, 2019. *MMWR Morbidity and Mortality Weekly Report, 71*(1), 1-9. https://doi.org/10.15585/mmwr.mm7101a1

Lee, Y. B., Yu, J., Choi, H. H., Jeon, B. S., Kim, H.-K., Kim, S.-W., Kim, S. S., Park, Y. G., & Chae, H. S. (2017). The association between peptic ulcer diseases and mental health problems. *Medicine, 96*(34), Article e7828. https://doi.org/10.1097/md.0000000000007828

Leeming, E. R., Johnson, A. J., Spector, T. D., & Le Roy, C. I. (2019). Effect of Diet on the Gut Microbiota: Rethinking Intervention Duration. *Nutrients, 11*(12), Article 2862. https://doi.org/10.3390/nu11122862

Leeuwendaal, N. K., Stanton, C., O'Toole, P. W., & Beresford, T. P. (2022). Fermented Foods, Health and the Gut Microbiome. *Nutrients, 14*(7), Article 1527. https://doi.org/10.3390/nu14071527

Leigh, S., Uhlig, F., Wilmes, L., Sanchez-Diaz, P., Gheorghe, C. E., Goodson, M. S., Kelley-Loughnane, N., Hyland, N. P., Cryan, J. F., & Clarke, G. (2023). The impact of acute and chronic stress on gastrointestinal physiology and function: a microbiota–gut–brain axis perspective. *The Journal of Physiology, 601*(20), 4491–4538. https://doi.org/10.1113/jp281951

Leone, V., Gibbons, S. M., Martinez, K., Hutchison, A. L., Huang, E. Y., Cham, C. M., Pierre, J. F., Heneghan, A. F., Nadimpalli, A., Hubert, N., Zale, E., Wang, Y., Huang, Y., Theriault, B., Dinner, A. R., Musch, M. W., Kudsk, K. A., Prendergast, B. J., Gilbert, J. A., & Chang, E. B. (2015). Effects of diurnal variation of gut microbes and high-fat feeding on host circadian clock function and metabolism. *Cell Host & Microbe*, *17*(5), 681–689. https://doi.org/10.1016/j.chom.2015.03.006

Lim, E. J., & Park, J. E. (2019). The effects of Pilates and yoga participant's on engagement in functional movement and individual health level. *Journal of Exercise Rehabilitation*, *15*(4), 553–559. https://doi.org/10.12965/jer.1938280.140

Mahmood, A., FitzGerald, A. J., Marchbank, T., Ntatsaki, E., Murray, D., Ghosh, S., & Playford, R. J. (2007). Zinc carnosine, a health food supplement that stabilises small bowel integrity and stimulates gut repair processes. *Gut*, *56*(2), 168–175. https://doi.org/10.1136/gut.2006.099929

Mahmud, Md. R., Akter, S., Tamanna, S. K., Mazumder, L., Esti, I. Z., Banerjee, S., Akter, S., Hasan, Md. R., Acharjee, M., Hossain, Md. S., & Pirttilä, A. M. (2022). Impact of gut microbiome on skin health: gut-skin axis observed through the lenses of therapeutics and skin diseases. *Gut Microbes*, *14*(1), Article 2096995. https://doi.org/10.1080/19490976.2022.2096995

Mar-Solís, L. M., Soto-Domínguez, A., Rodríguez-Tovar, L. E., Rodríguez-Rocha, H., García-García, A., Aguirre-Arzola, V. E., Zamora-Ávila, D. E., Garza-Arredondo, A. J., & Castillo-Velázquez, U. (2021). Analysis of the Anti-Inflammatory Capacity of Bone Broth in a Murine Model of Ulcerative Colitis. *Medicina*, *57*(11), 1138. https://doi.org/10.3390/medicina57111138

Martinez, K. B., Pierre, J. F., & Chang, E. B. (2016). The Gut Microbiota. *Gastroenterology Clinics of North America*, *45*(4), 601–614. https://doi.org/10.1016/j.gtc.2016.07.001

Mayo Clinic. (2023). *How much fiber is found in common foods?* Mayo Clinic. https://www.mayoclinic.org/healthy-lifestyle/nutrition-and-healthy-eating/in-depth/high-fiber-foods/art-20050948

McDonald, E. (2018, September 23). *A hot topic: Are spicy foods healthy or dangerous?* At the Forefront; UChicago Medicine. Retrieved January 24, 2024, https://www.uchicagomedicine.org/forefront/health-and-wellness-articles/spicy-foods-healthy-or-dangerous

McKeown, N. M., Fahey, G. C., Slavin, J., & van der Kamp, J.-W. (2022). Fibre Intake for Optimal Health: How Can Healthcare Professionals Support People to Reach Dietary Recommendations? *BMJ*, *378*, Article e054370. https://doi.org/10.1136/bmj-2020-054370

Monda, V., Villano, I., Messina, A., Valenzano, A., Esposito, T., Moscatelli, F., Viggiano, A., Cibelli, G., Chieffi, S., Monda, M., & Messina, G. (2017). Exercise

Modifies the Gut Microbiota with Positive Health Effects. *Oxidative Medicine and Cellular Longevity, 2017,* Article 3831972. https://doi.org/10.1155/2017/3831972

Nam, Y., Kwon, S.-C., Lee, Y.-J., Jang, E.-C., & Ahn, S. (2018). Relationship between job stress and functional dyspepsia in display manufacturing sector workers: a cross-sectional study. *Annals of Occupational and Environmental Medicine, 30*(1), Article 62. https://doi.org/10.1186/s40557-018-0274-4

National Center for Complementary and Integrative Health. (2022, June). *Meditation and Mindfulness: What You Need To Know.* NCCIH National Center for Complementary and Integrative Health. https://www.nccih.nih.gov/health/meditation-and-mindfulness-what-you-need-to-know

Nelson, J. B. (2017). Mindful Eating: The Art of Presence While You Eat. *Diabetes Spectrum, 30*(3), 171–174. https://doi.org/10.2337/ds17-0015

Newberry, C., & Lynch, K. (2019). The role of diet in the development and management of gastroesophageal reflux disease: why we feel the burn. *Journal of Thoracic Disease, 11*(S12), 1594–1601. https://doi.org/10.21037/jtd.2019.06.42

Nicklett, E. J., & Kadell, A. R. (2013). Fruit and vegetable intake among older adults: A scoping review. *Maturitas, 75*(4), 305–312. https://doi.org/10.1016/j.maturitas.2013.05.005

National University of Health Sciences (2018, December 5). *5 Health Issues You Didn't Know Could be Caused by Poor Gut Health.* National University of Health Sciences. Retrieved January 17, 2024, https://www.nuhs.edu/5-health-issues-you-didnt-know-could-be-caused-by-poor-gut-health

Ogobuiro, I., Tuma, F., Gonzales, J., & Shumway, K. (n.d.). *Physiology, Gastrointestinal.* National Library of Medicine; StatPearls Publishing. Retrieved January 26, 2024, https://www.ncbi.nlm.nih.gov/books/NBK537103

Peak Pilates. (n.d.). *Exercise Spotlight: Spine Stretch Forward.* Peak Pilates. Retrieved January 27, 2024, https://theteaser.peakpilates.com/exercise-spotlight-spine-stretch-forward

Perna, S., Alalwan, T. A., Alaali, Z., Alnashaba, T., Gasparri, C., Infantino, V., Hammad, L., Riva, A., Petrangolini, G., Allegrini, P., & Rondanelli, M. (2019). The Role of Glutamine in the Complex Interaction between Gut Microbiota and Health: A Narrative Review. *International Journal of Molecular Sciences, 20*(20), Article 5232. https://doi.org/10.3390/ijms20205232

Physitrack. (n.d.-a). *Step-by-step guide to Body Saws.* Physitrack. Retrieved January 27, 2024, https://www.physitrack.com/exercise-library/how-to-perform-the-body-saws

Physitrack. (n.d.-b). *Step-by-step guide to the the [sic] hundred in pilates exercise.* Physitrack. Retrieved January 27, 2024, https://www.physitrack.com/exercise-library/how-to-perform-the-the-hundred-in-pilates-exercise

Polhuis, K., Wijnen, A., Sierksma, A., Calame, W., & Tieland, M. (2017). The Diuretic Action of Weak and Strong Alcoholic Beverages in Elderly Men: A Randomized Diet-Controlled Crossover Trial. *Nutrients, 9*(7), Article 660. https://doi.org/10.3390/nu9070660

Popkin, B. M., D'Anci, K. E., & Rosenberg, I. H. (2020). Water, Hydration, and Health. *Nutrition Reviews, 68*(8), 439–458. https://doi.org/10.1111/j.1753-4887.2010.00304.x

Pouille, C. L., Ouaza, S., Roels, E., Behra, J., Tourret, M., Molinié, R., Fontaine, J.-X., Mathiron, D., Gagneul, D., Taminiau, B., Daube, G., Ravallec, R., Rambaud, C., Hilbert, J.-L., Cudennec, B., & Lucau-Danila, A. (2022). Chicory: Understanding the Effects and Effectors of This Functional Food. *Nutrients, 14*(5), Article 957. https://doi.org/10.3390/nu14050957

Qi, L. (2021). Fried Foods, Gut Microbiota, and Glucose Metabolism. *Diabetes Care, 44*(9), 1907–1909. https://doi.org/10.2337/dci21-0033

Reed, C. (2022, September 14). *New survey finds forty percent of Americans' daily lives are disrupted by digestive troubles*. American Gastroenterological Association. Retrieved January 24, 2024, https://gastro.org/press-releases/new-survey-finds-forty-percent-of-americans-daily-lives-are-disrupted-by-digestive-troubles

Ronis, M. J. J., Pedersen, K. B., & Watt, J. (2018). Adverse Effects of Nutraceuticals and Dietary Supplements. *Annual Review of Pharmacology and Toxicology, 58*(1), 583–601. https://doi.org/10.1146/annurev-pharmtox-010617-052844

Ruiz-Ojeda, F. J., Plaza-Díaz, J., Sáez-Lara, M. J., & Gil, A. (2019). Effects of Sweeteners on the Gut Microbiota: A Review of Experimental Studies and Clinical Trials. *Advances in Nutrition, 10*(suppl_1), S31–S48. https://doi.org/10.1093/advances/nmy037

Russo, M. A., Santarelli, D. M., & O'Rourke, D. (2017). The physiological effects of slow breathing in the healthy human. *Breathe, 13*(4), 298–309. https://doi.org/10.1183/20734735.009817

Rutsch, A., Kantsjö, J. B., & Ronchi, F. (2020). The Gut-Brain Axis: How Microbiota and Host Inflammasome Influence Brain Physiology and Pathology. *Frontiers in Immunology, 11*, Article 604179. https://doi.org/10.3389/fimmu.2020.604179

Scazzocchio, B., Minghetti, L., & D'Archivio, M. (2020). Interaction between Gut Microbiota and Curcumin: A New Key of Understanding for the Health Effects of Curcumin. *Nutrients, 12*(9), Article 2499. https://doi.org/10.3390/nu12092499

Seal, A. D., Bardis, C. N., Gavrieli, A., Grigorakis, P., Adams, J. D., Arnaoutis, G., Yannakoulia, M., & Kavouras, S. A. (2017). Coffee with High but Not Low Caffeine Content Augments Fluid and Electrolyte Excretion at Rest. *Frontiers in Nutrition, 4*(40). https://doi.org/10.3389/fnut.2017.00040

Shirreffs, S. M. (2009). Hydration in sport and exercise: water, sports drinks and other drinks. *Nutrition Bulletin, 34*(4), 374–379. https://doi.org/10.1111/j.1467-3010.2009.01790.x

Shurney, D. (2019). The Gut Microbiome: Unleashing the Doctor Within. *American Journal of Lifestyle Medicine, 13*(3), 265–268. https://doi.org/10.1177/1559827619826551

Sievers, M. (2021, September 28). *The Pilates Bridge | Tutorials, Benefits, and Progressions*. Pilates Encyclopedia. Retrieved January 27, 2024, https://www.pilatesencyclopedia.com/blog/bridging

Singh, R., Zogg, H., Wei, L., Bartlett, A., Ghoshal, U. C., Rajender, S., & Ro, S. (2020). Gut Microbial Dysbiosis in the Pathogenesis of Gastrointestinal Dysmotility and Metabolic Disorders. *Journal of Neurogastroenterology and Motility, 27*(1), 19–34. https://doi.org/10.5056/jnm20149

Song, E. M., Jung, H.-K., & Jung, J. M. (2012). The Association Between Reflux Esophagitis and Psychosocial Stress. *Digestive Diseases and Sciences, 58*(2), 471–477. https://doi.org/10.1007/s10620-012-2377-z

Song, X., Zhang, X., Ma, C., Hu, X., & Chen, F. (2022). Rediscovering the nutrition of whole foods: the emerging role of gut microbiota. *Current Opinion in Food Science, 48*, Article 100908. https://doi.org/10.1016/j.cofs.2022.100908

Stengel, A., & Taché, Y. (2009). Neuroendocrine Control of the Gut During Stress: Corticotropin-Releasing Factor Signaling Pathways in the Spotlight. *Annual Review of Physiology, 71*(1), 219–239. https://doi.org/10.1146/annurev.physiol.010908.163221

Tavoian, D., & Craighead, D. H. (2023). Deep breathing exercise at work: Potential applications and impact. *Frontiers in Physiology, 14*, Article 1040091. https://doi.org/10.3389/fphys.2023.1040091

Taylor, V. (2023, September). *What are whole foods?* Heart Matters. British Heart Foundation. Retrieved January 24, 2024, https://www.bhf.org.uk/information support/heart-matters-magazine/nutrition/whole-foods

Thompson, S. V., Bailey, M. A., Taylor, A. M., Kaczmarek, J. L., Mysonhimer, A. R., Edwards, C. G., Reeser, G. E., Burd, N. A., Khan, N. A., & Holscher, H. D. (2021). Avocado Consumption Alters Gastrointestinal Bacteria Abundance and Microbial Metabolite Concentrations among Adults with Overweight or Obesity: A Randomized Controlled Trial. *The Journal of Nutrition, 151*(4), 753–762. https://doi.org/10.1093/jn/nxaa219

Thursby, E., & Juge, N. (2017). Introduction to the human gut microbiota. *Biochemical Journal, 474*(11), 1823–1836. https://doi.org/10.1042/bcj20160510

Tindle, J., & Tadi, P. (n.d.). *Neuroanatomy, Parasympathetic Nervous System*. National Library of Medicine; StatPearls Publishing. Retrieved January 27, 2024, https://www.ncbi.nlm.nih.gov/books/NBK553141

UCSF Health. (n.d.). *Increasing Fiber Intake*. The University of California San Francisco. Retrieved January 27, 2024, https://www.ucsfhealth.org/education/increasing-fiber-intake

US Department of Agriculture. (n.d.). *FoodData Central*. U.S. Department of Agriculture. Retrieved January 27, 2024, https://fdc.nal.usda.gov

Vanhaecke, T., Bretin, O., Poirel, M., & Tap, J. (2022). Drinking Water Source and Intake Are Associated with Distinct Gut Microbiota Signatures in US and UK Populations. *The Journal of Nutrition*, *152*(1), 171–182. https://doi.org/10.1093/jn/nxab312

Vetrani, C., Di Nisio, A., Paschou, S. A., Barrea, L., Muscogiuri, G., Graziadio, C., Savastano, S., & Colao, A. (2022). From Gut Microbiota through Low-Grade Inflammation to Obesity: Key Players and Potential Targets. *Nutrients*, *14*(10), Article 2103. https://doi.org/10.3390/nu14102103

von Duvillard, S. P., Braun, W. A., Markofski, M., Beneke, R., & Leithäuser, R. (2004). Fluids and hydration in prolonged endurance performance. *Nutrition*, *20*(7-8), 651–656. https://doi.org/10.1016/j.nut.2004.04.011

Walker, C. (2015). *The Effects of an American Diet on Health*. Inquiro - Journal of Undergrad Research - Volume 9; The University of Alabama at Birmingham. Retrieved January 24, 2024, https://www.uab.edu/inquiro/issues/past-issues/volume-9/the-effects-of-an-american-diet-on-health

Wang, X., Zhang, D., Jiang, H., Zhang, S., Pang, X., Gao, S., Zhang, H., Zhang, S., Xiao, Q., Chen, L., Wang, S., Qi, D., & Li, Y. (2021). Gut Microbiota Variation With Short-Term Intake of Ginger Juice on Human Health. *Frontiers in Microbiology*, *11*, Article 576061. https://doi.org/10.3389/fmicb.2020.576061

Wang, Y., Uffelman, C. N., Bergia, R. E., Clark, C. M., Reed, J. B., Cross, T.-W. L., Lindemann, S. R., Tang, M., & Campbell, W. W. (2023). Meat Consumption and Gut Microbiota: a Scoping Review of Literature and Systematic Review of Randomized Controlled Trials in Adults. *Advances in Nutrition*, *14*(2), 215–237. https://doi.org/10.1016/j.advnut.2022.10.005

Watts, G. (n.d.). *Anatomy of the Perfect Pilates Roll Up Exercise: Tips and Tricks*. Pilates Lesson Planner. Retrieved January 24, 2024, https://pilateslessonplans.co.uk/anatomy-of-the-perfect-pilates-roll-up-exercise

Witek, K., Wydra, K., & Filip, M. (2022). A High-Sugar Diet Consumption, Metabolism and Health Impacts with a Focus on the Development of Substance Use Disorder: A Narrative Review. *Nutrients*, *14*(14), Article 2940. https://doi.org/10.3390/nu14142940

Wu, J., Zhang, B., Zhou, S., Huang, Z., Xu, Y., Lu, X., Zheng, X., & Ouyang, D. (2023). Associations between gut microbiota and sleep: a two-sample, bidirectional Mendelian randomization study. *Frontiers in Microbiology*, *14*, Article 1236847. https://doi.org/10.3389/fmicb.2023.1236847

Xiong, R.-G., Li, J., Cheng, J., Zhou, D.-D., Wu, S.-X., Huang, S.-Y., Saimaiti, A., Yang, Z.-J., Gan, R.-Y., & Li, H.-B. (2023). The Role of Gut Microbiota in Anxiety, Depression, and Other Mental Disorders as Well as the Protective Effects of Dietary Components. *Nutrients*, *15*(14), Article 3258. https://doi.org/10.3390/nu15143258

Yoo, J., Groer, M., Dutra, S., Sarkar, A., & McSkimming, D. (2020). Gut Microbiota and Immune System Interactions. *Microorganisms*, *8*(10), Article 1587. https://doi.org/10.3390/microorganisms8101587

Youssef, M., Ahmed, H. Y., Zongo, A., Korin, A., Zhan, F., Hady, E., Umair, M., Shahid Riaz Rajoka, M., Xiong, Y., & Li, B. (2021). Probiotic Supplements: Their Strategies in the Therapeutic and Prophylactic of Human Life-Threatening Diseases. *International Journal of Molecular Sciences*, *22*(20), Article 11290. https://doi.org/10.3390/ijms222011290

Zhang, M., & Yang, X.-J. (2016). Effects of a high fat diet on intestinal microbiota and gastrointestinal diseases. *World Journal of Gastroenterology*, *22*(40), Article 8905. https://doi.org/10.3748/wjg.v22.i40.8905

www.ingramcontent.com/pod-product-compliance
Lightning Source LLC
LaVergne TN
LVHW040101080526
838202LV00045B/3722